The Late Adult Autism Diagnosis Handbook

A Practical Guide to Self-Discovery, Understanding, Unmasking, and Thriving After a Later-in-Life Autism Diagnosis

Carlo Faron Oneal

Copyright Notice

The Late Adult Autism Diagnosis Handbook

Copyright © 2025 by Carlo Faron Oneal

All rights reserved. No part of this publication may be reproduced, distributed, or transmitted in any form or by any means, including photocopying, recording, digital scanning, or other electronic or mechanical methods, without the prior written permission of the publisher, except in the case of brief quotations embodied in critical reviews and certain other noncommercial uses permitted by copyright law.

ISBN: 978-1-7641438-8-2

Isohan Publishing

First Edition: 2025

Disclaimer

Medical and Professional Disclaimer

The information contained in this book is for general educational and informational purposes only. It is not intended as, and should not be understood or construed as, professional medical, psychological, psychiatric, or other healthcare advice. The content is not intended to be a substitute for professional diagnosis, treatment, or advice.

Always seek the advice of your physician, mental health professional, or other qualified health provider with any questions you may have regarding autism spectrum disorder or any medical condition. Never disregard professional medical advice or delay in seeking it because of something you have read in this book.

The author and publisher are not responsible for any adverse effects or consequences resulting from the use of any suggestions, preparations, or procedures described in this book.

Legal and Accommodation Disclaimer

While this book discusses legal rights and workplace/educational accommodations, laws and regulations vary significantly by jurisdiction and change over time. The legal information provided is general in nature and may not apply to your specific situation or location. This book does not constitute legal advice. For legal matters, please consult with a qualified attorney familiar with disability law in your jurisdiction.

Personal Experience Disclaimer

The strategies, techniques, and approaches described in this book are based on current research, clinical practices, and the experiences of many autistic adults. However, every individual on the autism spectrum is unique. What works for one person may not work for another. The author encourages readers to adapt the information to their own specific needs and circumstances.

Case Studies and Examples

The names and scenarios depicted in this book are purely for illustrative purposes only. Any resemblance to actual persons, living or dead, or actual events is purely coincidental.

All case studies, examples, and personal stories presented in this book have been created as composite illustrations drawn from common experiences in the autistic community. Names, identifying details, and specific circumstances have been changed or combined to protect privacy and confidentiality. These examples are intended to illustrate typical challenges and experiences faced by late-diagnosed autistic adults but should not be taken as representing any specific individual's experience.

Resources and Links

While every effort has been made to ensure that the information regarding organizations, websites, and resources mentioned in this book was correct at the time of publication, the author and publisher do not assume and hereby disclaim any liability for the accuracy, completeness, or continued availability of such resources. Websites and organizations may change their focus, cease operations, or modify their services without notice.

Limitation of Liability

In no event shall the author or publisher be liable for any special, incidental, indirect, or consequential damages whatsoever arising out of or in connection with your use of or reliance on the information contained in this book.

Final Note

This book is intended to be a helpful resource for adults navigating late autism diagnosis. It represents the author's interpretation of current research and community knowledge at the time of writing. The field of autism research is rapidly evolving, and understanding continues to develop. Readers are encouraged to seek out the most current information and to connect with the autistic community for ongoing support and updated perspectives.

By using this book, you acknowledge that you have read and understood this disclaimer and agree to be bound by its terms.

Table of Contents

Chapter 1: What is Autism Spectrum Disorder? 1
Defining Autism Beyond Stereotypes 1
The Spectrum Concept Explained 2
Neurodiversity Perspective vs. Medical Model 3
Common Myths About Autism Debunked 5
Chapter FAQ: "Is autism really a spectrum?" 6
Key Takeaways 8

Chapter 2: Why Autism Goes Undiagnosed Until Adulthood 9
Historical Diagnostic Criteria and Its Evolution 9
Gender Bias in Diagnosis 10
Cultural Factors Affecting Recognition 12
The "Lost Generation" of Undiagnosed Adults 13
How Autism Presents Differently Across the Lifespan 15
FAQ: "Why wasn't I diagnosed as a child?" 17

Chapter 3: Adult Autism Presentation 20
Masking and Camouflaging Behaviors 20
Compensatory Strategies Developed Over Time 22
Executive Function Challenges in Adult Life 24
Sensory Differences in Adult Contexts 26
Social Communication in Professional Settings 27
FAQ: "How do I know if I'm masking?" 30
Key Takeaways 31

Chapter 4: Self-Discovery and Pre-Diagnosis 33

    Common Paths to Self-Identification............................33
    Online Assessments and Screening Tools 35
    Building Your Case History...37
    Documenting Childhood Experiences..........................39
    Preparing for Professional Assessment 40
    Chapter FAQ: "Should I self-diagnose?"......................42
    Key Takeaways 43

Chapter 5: Getting a Professional Diagnosis................. 45
    Finding Qualified Diagnosticians 45
    Types of Assessments Available...................................47
    What to Expect During Evaluation...............................49
    Cost Considerations and Insurance 51
    International Differences in Diagnostic Processes 53
    Chapter FAQ: "How much does diagnosis cost?" 55
    Key Takeaways 56
    Crossing the Threshold 57

Chapter 6: After Your Diagnosis 58
    Processing the Diagnosis Emotionally 58
    Identity Reconstruction 60
    Dealing with Imposter Syndrome 62
    Sharing Your Diagnosis Strategically 64
    Building Your Support Team 66
    FAQ: "Do I have to tell everyone?" 69
    Key Takeaways 70
    The Journey Continues 70

Chapter 7: Workplace Rights and Accommodations 72
Legal Protections (ADA, Equivalent Laws Globally)....... 72
Reasonable Accommodation Examples 74
Disclosure Decisions and Scripts 76
Self-Advocacy Strategies 78
Career Considerations 80
FAQ: "Should I tell my employer?" 83
Key Takeaways 84
Preparing for Academic Success 85

Chapter 8: Educational Accommodations 86
Rights in Higher Education 86
Accommodation Request Process 88
Study Strategies for Autistic Learners 91
Managing Academic Stress 94
Online Learning Considerations 96
FAQ: "Can I get accommodations without formal diagnosis?" 98
Key Takeaways 100
Healthcare Navigation Ahead 100

Chapter 9: Healthcare and Therapy Options 101
Finding Autism-Informed Providers 101
Therapy Approaches (CBT Adaptations, DBT) 104
Occupational Therapy for Adults 107
Managing Co-occurring Conditions 110
Medication Considerations 112

Chapter FAQ: "Do I need therapy if I'm doing fine?" 115

Key Takeaways 117

Building Daily Living Skills 117

Chapter 10: Daily Living Strategies 119

Executive Function Supports 119

Sensory Management Techniques 122

Energy Management and Burnout Prevention 126

Home Environment Modifications 129

Technology Tools and Apps 131

FAQ: "How do I prevent autistic burnout?" 133

Chapter 11: Relationships and Communication 137

Explaining Autism to Family and Friends 137

Dating and Romantic Relationships 139

Parenting as an Autistic Adult 143

Friendship Maintenance Strategies 145

Setting Boundaries 146

Chapter FAQ: "How do I explain my needs to my partner?" 148

Key Takeaways 150

Building Community Connections 150

Chapter 12: Finding Your Community 151

Online Autistic Communities 151

Local Support Groups 153

Advocacy Organizations 156

Peer Mentorship Programs 158

Building Chosen Family 160

   Chapter FAQ: "Where do I find other autistic adults?" .. 161

   Key Takeaways 163

Chapter 13: Reframing Your Past 164

   Understanding Your Life Through an Autistic Lens 164

   Healing from Misdiagnosis and Trauma 166

   Celebrating Autistic Strengths 169

   Letting Go of Shame 171

   Writing Your New Narrative 173

   Chapter FAQ: "How do I stop feeling broken?" 174

   Key Takeaways 175

   Building Your Future 176

Chapter 14: Future Planning 177

   Long-term Support Needs 177

   Financial Planning Considerations 180

   Healthcare Directives 182

   Building Sustainable Routines 184

   Advocacy and Giving Back 186

   Chapter FAQ: "What does my future look like?" 188

   Key Takeaways 190

   Your Handbook Continues 190

Appendix A: Diagnostic Worksheets 192

   Childhood History Questionnaire 192

   Current Challenges Inventory 195

   Sensory Profile Worksheet 197

  Communication Preferences Chart 199

Appendix B: Communication Scripts 202
  Disclosure Scripts for Various Situations 202
  Accommodation Request Templates 204
  Boundary-Setting Phrases 206
  Medical Appointment Preparation 207

Appendix C: Resources Directory 209
  Professional Organizations 209
  Online Communities 210
  Recommended Books and Websites 211
  Apps and Tools 212
  Crisis Resources 212

Appendix D: Quick Reference Guides 214
  Common Autistic Traits Checklist 214
  Masking Behaviors Identifier 215
  Burnout Warning Signs 216
  Self-Advocacy Tips 217
  Sensory Regulation Techniques 218

Glossary of Terms 220
  A 220
  B 223
  C 224
  D 227
  E 229
  F 230

G	231
H	232
I	233
J	234
K	234
L	235
M	236
N	237
O	238
P	238
Q	240
R	240
S	241
T	244
U	246
V	246
W	247
X	247
Y	247
Z	248
References	**249**

Chapter 1: What is Autism Spectrum Disorder?

The human brain processes information in countless ways, and autism represents one of many natural variations in how people experience and interact with the world. For decades, society has misunderstood autism, building walls of misconception that have left millions of adults wondering why they've always felt different. Understanding autism spectrum disorder (ASD) requires looking past the outdated stereotypes and recognizing it as a neurological difference that affects communication, sensory processing, social interaction, and behavior patterns.

Defining Autism Beyond Stereotypes

Autism spectrum disorder encompasses a broad range of experiences, abilities, and challenges that vary significantly from person to person. The diagnostic criteria focus on differences in social communication and interaction, along with restricted or repetitive patterns of behavior, interests, or activities (1). Yet these clinical definitions barely scratch the surface of what it means to be autistic.

Consider Sarah, a 42-year-old marketing executive who recently discovered she's autistic. Throughout her career, she excelled at data analysis and pattern recognition, often spotting trends her colleagues missed. She structured her days meticulously, arriving at the office at exactly 7:47 AM and eating the same lunch at her desk while reviewing spreadsheets. Her coworkers saw her as quirky but brilliant. What they didn't see was how she rehearsed every meeting interaction the night before, how fluorescent lights made her skin feel like it was burning, or how she needed two hours of complete silence after work to recover from the sensory assault of her open-plan office.

The stereotypical image of autism—often portrayed as a young, white male who struggles with eye contact and rocks back and forth—represents only a tiny fraction of the autistic experience. Many autistic adults, particularly those diagnosed later in life, have developed sophisticated coping mechanisms that mask their autistic traits. They might maintain eye contact despite discomfort, engage in small talk they find meaningless, or suppress their need for routine in social situations (2).

James, diagnosed at 38, spent years forcing himself to attend after-work social events, despite feeling physically ill from the noise and unpredictability. He learned to mirror his colleagues' body language and memorized appropriate responses to common social scenarios. His autism wasn't less real because he could "pass" as neurotypical—it simply meant he was expending enormous energy to appear typical while his authentic self remained hidden.

The Spectrum Concept Explained

The term "spectrum" in autism spectrum disorder often leads to misunderstanding. Many people envision a linear scale from "less autistic" to "more autistic," but this oversimplification fails to capture autism's multidimensional nature. Instead, think of the spectrum as a color wheel, where each person's profile includes varying intensities of different traits (3).

An autistic person might have exceptional verbal abilities but struggle with motor coordination. Another might process visual information at genius levels while finding spoken language challenging. Some autistic people need minimal support in daily life, while others require substantial assistance. Support needs can also fluctuate—the same person might function independently most days but need significant help during periods of stress or sensory overload.

Maria, a 35-year-old teacher, exemplifies this complexity. She delivers engaging lectures and connects deeply with students who struggle academically. Her ability to explain concepts in multiple ways comes from her own non-linear thinking patterns. However, she cannot tolerate the texture of most foods, eating only five specific meals in rotation. She excels at reading student emotions but misses social cues from colleagues. During parent-teacher conferences, she performs well for the first few meetings but becomes increasingly overwhelmed as the evening progresses, eventually losing the ability to speak coherently—a phenomenon known as selective mutism that affects some autistic people under stress (4).

The spectrum encompasses variations in:

- **Communication styles**: From non-speaking individuals who communicate through AAC devices to hyperverbal people who infodump about special interests
- **Sensory processing**: Ranging from sensory-seeking behaviors to extreme sensory avoidance
- **Social preferences**: Including those who crave connection but struggle with implementation to those genuinely preferring solitude
- **Executive function**: From individuals with exceptional organizational abilities in specific areas to those who struggle with basic daily planning
- **Motor skills**: Including both fine and gross motor differences
- **Information processing**: From detail-focused thinking to pattern recognition abilities

Neurodiversity Perspective vs. Medical Model

Two primary frameworks exist for understanding autism: the medical model and the neurodiversity paradigm. The medical model views autism as a disorder requiring treatment or cure, focusing on deficits and abnormalities. This perspective dominated autism research and intervention for decades, leading to therapies aimed at making autistic people appear more neurotypical (5).

The neurodiversity movement, pioneered by autistic advocates, reframes autism as a natural variation in human neurology rather than a pathology requiring correction (6). This perspective acknowledges that while autistic people may need support and accommodations, their different way of processing the world isn't inherently inferior. Just as biodiversity strengthens ecosystems, neurodiversity enriches human communities.

Consider how these perspectives might view common autistic traits:

Medical Model View:

- Restricted interests = obsessive behavior requiring intervention
- Sensory sensitivities = sensory processing disorder needing therapy
- Direct communication = social skills deficit
- Need for routine = inflexibility requiring treatment

Neurodiversity View:

- Focused interests = passion and expertise development
- Sensory differences = unique perceptual experiences requiring accommodation
- Direct communication = honest, efficient interaction style
- Need for routine = effective anxiety management and productivity strategy

Dr. Chen, diagnosed at 45, found the neurodiversity framework transformative. The medical model had labeled his intense focus on cardiac surgery techniques as "perseveration." Through a neurodiversity lens, this same trait made him an exceptional surgeon who developed innovative procedures. His need for specific surgical tools arranged in exact patterns wasn't rigidity—it was optimization that improved patient outcomes.

Neither framework tells the complete story. Many autistic adults find value in both perspectives, using the medical model to access needed supports while embracing neurodiversity principles for self-acceptance and advocacy. The key lies in recognizing that autism involves real challenges requiring support while rejecting the notion that autistic people are broken versions of neurotypical people (7).

Common Myths About Autism Debunked

Persistent myths about autism create barriers to recognition, especially for adults seeking diagnosis. Let's examine and dispel the most harmful misconceptions:

Myth 1: Autistic people lack empathy Reality: Autistic people often experience intense empathy but may express it differently. The "double empathy problem" shows that communication difficulties go both ways—neurotypical people struggle to understand autistic experiences just as much as autistic people struggle with neurotypical social norms (8). Many autistic individuals report feeling others' emotions so intensely that they become overwhelming, leading to shutdown or withdrawal that gets misinterpreted as lack of caring.

Myth 2: Autism is a childhood condition Reality: Autism is a lifelong neurological difference. Children don't "grow out of" autism, though they may develop coping strategies that mask their traits. Many adults remain undiagnosed because diagnostic criteria historically focused on how autism presents in young boys, missing how it manifests in adults, women, and people of color (9).

Myth 3: All autistic people have intellectual disabilities
Reality: Autism occurs across all intelligence levels. While some autistic people have intellectual disabilities, many have average or above-average intelligence. The association stems from communication differences being misinterpreted as cognitive limitations and from IQ tests that don't accommodate autistic learning styles (10).

Myth 4: Autistic people don't want social relationships
Reality: Social motivation varies among autistic people just as it does among neurotypicals. Many autistic adults deeply desire connection but struggle with neurotypical social conventions. They may prefer smaller gatherings, need recovery time after socializing, or connect better through shared interests than small talk (11).

Myth 5: You can't be autistic if you're married/have a job/went to college Reality: Autistic people achieve all these milestones. They may accomplish them differently—perhaps taking longer to complete college due to executive function challenges, choosing careers that align with their interests and sensory needs, or finding partners who appreciate direct communication. Success doesn't negate the need for support or the reality of being autistic (12).

Myth 6: Autism is caused by vaccines/parenting/diet Reality: Autism is a hereditable neurological variation present from birth. The vaccine myth has been thoroughly debunked by extensive research. While environmental factors may influence how autism presents, the fundamental neurological differences are genetic. Parent-blaming theories caused immense harm to families and delayed recognition of autism's true nature (13).

Chapter FAQ: "Is autism really a spectrum?"

Yes, autism is genuinely a spectrum, but not in the linear "mild to severe" way many people imagine. Think of it more like a sound mixing board with dozens of sliders, each representing different aspects of the autistic experience. Each person's unique combination of settings creates their individual autistic profile.

The spectrum includes variations in:

- **Communication abilities**: From non-speaking to hyperverbal
- **Sensory processing**: Across all senses with varying sensitivities
- **Executive function**: Different abilities in planning, organizing, and task switching
- **Social processing**: Varied abilities and preferences for social interaction
- **Motor skills**: Range of fine and gross motor abilities
- **Information processing styles**: From detail-focused to pattern-recognition
- **Support needs**: Fluctuating based on environment, stress, and life demands

Support needs don't correlate neatly with abilities. A university professor might need minimal support at work but require assistance with daily living tasks. A non-speaking person might have profound insights they share through writing. Someone who appears to cope well might be masking at enormous personal cost.

The spectrum concept recognizes that autism isn't better or worse at different "points"—it's simply different combinations of traits. Each autistic person has their own profile of strengths, challenges, abilities, and support needs that can change throughout their life and across different contexts.

Key Takeaways

- Autism is a neurological variation affecting communication, sensory processing, social interaction, and behavior patterns—not a disease or deficit
- The autism spectrum represents multidimensional variations in traits rather than a linear scale from "mild" to "severe"
- Both medical model and neurodiversity perspectives offer valuable insights for understanding and supporting autistic experiences
- Common myths about autism create barriers to recognition and acceptance, particularly for adults seeking diagnosis
- Every autistic person has a unique profile of abilities, challenges, and support needs that may fluctuate based on context and life circumstances
- Understanding autism requires moving beyond stereotypes to recognize the full diversity of autistic experiences

Chapter 2: Why Autism Goes Undiagnosed Until Adulthood

Thousands of adults are discovering they're autistic in their 30s, 40s, 50s, and beyond. This isn't a new phenomenon—these individuals were autistic all along. What's new is our expanding understanding of how autism presents across different populations and life stages. The journey to late diagnosis often involves years of misunderstandings, misdiagnoses, and the exhausting work of trying to fit into a world that feels fundamentally misaligned with your operating system.

Historical Diagnostic Criteria and Its Evolution

The diagnostic criteria for autism have undergone radical transformation since Leo Kanner first described "infantile autism" in 1943 (14). Kanner's original cases included only children with significant support needs who showed obvious differences from typical development. Around the same time, Hans Asperger described children with similar social communication differences but strong language abilities—though his work remained largely unknown in English-speaking countries until the 1980s (15).

For decades, autism diagnosis required evidence of differences before age three, effectively excluding anyone whose traits became apparent later or whose early differences went unnoticed. The criteria focused heavily on observable behaviors in young children, particularly:

- Language delays or absence
- Obvious repetitive behaviors like hand-flapping or rocking
- Apparent lack of interest in others
- Absence of imaginative play

These criteria missed countless children who developed compensatory strategies, whose special interests aligned with gender expectations, or whose families adapted around their needs without recognizing them as unusual.

Robert, now 52, exemplifies this diagnostic gap. As a child in the 1970s, he lined up his toy cars in perfect color gradients, ate only beige foods, and recited entire encyclopedia entries about trains. His parents called him "quirky" and "gifted." His teachers noted his difficulty with group work but praised his exceptional memory. When he covered his ears during fire drills, adults told him to "stop being dramatic." No one considered autism because he spoke in full sentences by age two and made eye contact when reminded.

The DSM-III in 1980 introduced "Infantile Autism" as an official diagnosis, but the criteria remained restrictive. The DSM-IV in 1994 added Asperger's Syndrome, finally acknowledging that autism could exist without language delays or intellectual disabilities (16). However, this created an artificial divide between "high-functioning" and "low-functioning" autism that many advocates now reject as harmful and inaccurate.

The DSM-5 in 2013 consolidated all autism-related diagnoses into Autism Spectrum Disorder, recognizing autism as a single condition with varied presentations (17). Significantly, it removed the requirement for symptoms to be present before age three, instead stating that traits must be present in early development but may not fully manifest until social demands exceed capacities. This change opened the door for adult diagnosis, acknowledging that autism might be masked, compensated for, or simply missed in childhood.

Gender Bias in Diagnosis

Perhaps no factor has contributed more to missed diagnoses than the pervasive gender bias in autism research and clinical practice. Early autism research focused almost exclusively on boys, establishing a diagnostic prototype that missed how autism presents in girls, women, and gender-diverse individuals (18).

The stereotypical autistic presentation—focused on trains or numbers, overtly struggling with social interaction, displaying obvious stimming behaviors—reflects how autism often presents in boys socialized in Western cultures. Girls are frequently socialized to mask their differences, leading to what researchers now call the "camouflage effect" (19).

Consider these gendered differences in presentation:

Common "male" presentations (though not exclusive to males):

- Special interests in objects, systems, or mechanics
- More overt social communication struggles
- Externalizing behaviors when overwhelmed
- Less social motivation for masking

Common "female" presentations (though not exclusive to females):

- Special interests in people, animals, or fiction
- Intense observation and mimicry of social behaviors
- Internalizing distress through anxiety or eating disorders
- High social motivation leading to exhaustive masking

Emma's story illustrates this perfectly. Throughout childhood, she collected facts about horses with encyclopedic detail, reading every horse book in the library multiple times. Unlike her male cousin's train obsession, adults saw her horse interest as typical for girls. She studied her classmates like an anthropologist, creating mental flowcharts of appropriate responses. By high school, she could perform "normal teenager" convincingly, though it left her depleted. Her meltdowns happened privately—sobbing in bathroom stalls or scratching her arms raw under her sleeves. Teachers called her "anxious" and "perfectionist," never considering autism.

The diagnostic gender gap has serious consequences. Studies suggest that autistic women and girls receive diagnoses an average of 4-5 years later than males (20). Many aren't diagnosed until their own children are assessed for autism, suddenly recognizing themselves in the diagnostic criteria. Others reach diagnosis through mental health crises, after years of misdiagnoses including:

- Borderline personality disorder
- Eating disorders
- Anxiety disorders
- Depression
- Bipolar disorder
- ADHD (though ADHD and autism frequently co-occur)

Trans and non-binary individuals face additional barriers, as gender dysphoria and autism can interplay in complex ways that many clinicians don't understand (21). The intersection of gender diversity and neurodiversity remains under-researched, leaving many people without appropriate support.

Cultural Factors Affecting Recognition

Culture profoundly shapes how autism presents and whether it gets recognized. Different cultures have varying expectations for eye contact, social interaction, emotional expression, and behavioral conformity—all areas affected by autism (22). What appears atypical in one culture might be unremarkable in another.

In many Asian cultures, for example, avoiding direct eye contact with authority figures shows respect rather than indicating a social communication difference. Quiet, studious behavior that might prompt autism evaluation in North America could be praised as ideal in educational systems that value conformity and academic focus. This cultural lens means autistic traits might be interpreted as positive character traits rather than neurological differences requiring support.

Marcus, a Black autistic man diagnosed at 41, describes how racial stereotypes obscured his autism throughout his life. His teachers interpreted his communication style as "defiance" rather than literal thinking. His need for clear, explicit instructions was seen as "challenging authority." When overwhelmed in class, his shutdowns were punished as "attitude problems." The school-to-prison pipeline nearly claimed him before a college professor recognized his behaviors as autistic traits and suggested evaluation (23).

Latino families might attribute autistic behaviors to "nervios" (nerves) or being "mal criado" (badly raised), leading to shame and hidden struggles rather than support-seeking. Indigenous communities might have traditional roles that accommodate autistic traits, but lose these protective factors through colonization and forced assimilation (24).

Diagnostic tools themselves carry cultural bias. Most autism assessments were developed using white, middle-class populations and may not accurately capture autism in people from different cultural backgrounds. Questions about play behaviors assume access to specific toys. Social communication assessments privilege Western conversation styles. Sensory questions might miss cultural differences in food, touch, or environmental stimuli.

The "Lost Generation" of Undiagnosed Adults

Millions of autistic adults born before the 1990s represent a "lost generation"—autistic people who reached adulthood without recognition or support for their neurological differences. They navigated education, employment, and relationships without understanding why everything felt harder for them than for their peers (25).

This generation developed elaborate coping mechanisms through trial and error:

- Creating rigid routines that others saw as "Type A personality"
- Choosing careers that minimized social demands
- Self-medicating with alcohol or drugs to manage sensory overload
- Developing anxiety or depression from constant masking
- Experiencing autistic burnout from unsustainable coping strategies

Jennifer, diagnosed at 58, spent four decades in survival mode. She chose night-shift nursing to avoid daytime social demands and sensory chaos. She memorized scripts for patient interactions and developed elaborate systems for managing medical charts. Her colleagues called her "detail-oriented" and "dedicated," never knowing she spent her days off in complete silence, recovering from the effort of appearing neurotypical. Three divorces later—each husband complaining she was "cold" and "inflexible"—she finally understood why relationships felt like performing in a foreign language.

Many from this generation reached diagnosis through their children or grandchildren. Watching a child's autism evaluation, they recognize their own experiences in the diagnostic criteria. Others find diagnosis after retirement, when the structure of work disappears and they can no longer maintain their coping mechanisms.

The lost generation often struggles with internalized ableism and identity reconstruction. After decades of being told they're "lazy," "weird," "difficult," or "broken," accepting themselves as autistic requires profound psychological work. They may grieve for the support they never received while celebrating finally understanding themselves.

How Autism Presents Differently Across the Lifespan

Autism doesn't look the same at 5, 25, 45, or 65. The core neurological differences remain consistent, but their expression changes with development, life experiences, and environmental demands (26). Understanding these lifespan variations helps explain why many autistic adults weren't diagnosed as children.

Early Childhood Presentation: Young autistic children might show:

- Sensory seeking or avoiding behaviors
- Intense interests in specific topics
- Echolalia or unique language development
- Preference for parallel play over interactive play
- Strong reactions to routine changes

However, in supportive environments with understanding caregivers, these traits might not cause significant distress or impairment—a requirement for diagnosis.

School Age Adaptations: As social demands increase, autistic children often develop masking strategies:

- Mimicking peer behaviors
- Suppressing stims in public
- Creating social "rules" through observation
- Channeling interests into acceptable academic pursuits

Academic success can mask struggles, especially for intellectually gifted autistic children who compensate through intelligence.

Adolescent Challenges: Puberty often represents a crisis point where previously effective coping strategies fail:

- Complex social dynamics become overwhelming
- Sensory sensitivities may intensify
- Identity formation conflicts with masking
- Mental health issues emerge from sustained stress

Many autistic teens experience their first major burnout during this period, though it might be misattributed to "teenage angst."

Adult Presentations: Autistic adults often show different patterns than children:

- Sophisticated masking strategies that hide obvious traits
- Careers chosen to accommodate sensory and social needs
- Relationships structured around autistic needs
- Burnout cycles from unsustainable coping
- Co-occurring mental health conditions from chronic stress

David's progression illustrates these changes. As a young child, he flapped his hands when excited and lined up toys. By elementary school, he learned to squeeze his fists instead of flapping and collected baseball cards—a more socially acceptable form of organizing objects. In high school, he memorized social rules and joined drama club to practice "performing normal." As an adult software developer, he channeled his pattern recognition into coding, structured his life to minimize sensory stressors, and maintained exactly three friendships through shared gaming interests. Only when his first child showed similar traits did he recognize his lifelong autism.

Later Life Considerations: Aging autistic adults face unique challenges:

- Loss of routine through retirement
- Sensory changes affecting established coping strategies
- Social isolation as masking becomes harder to maintain
- Misinterpretation of autistic traits as dementia
- Need for autism-informed elder care

FAQ: "Why wasn't I diagnosed as a child?"

Multiple factors likely contributed to your missed diagnosis:

1. **Diagnostic criteria limitations**: Until recently, criteria focused on young boys with obvious support needs. If you spoke on time, made any eye contact, or showed imaginative play, autism was ruled out.
2. **Successful masking**: You likely developed coping strategies that hid your autistic traits. What looked like shyness, anxiety, or quirkiness was actually autism masked through enormous effort.
3. **Gender bias**: If you're female or gender-diverse, diagnostic tools weren't designed to recognize your presentation. Your special interests might have seemed gender-typical, your social struggles attributed to other causes.
4. **Cultural factors**: Your family's cultural background might have interpreted autistic traits differently, or diagnostic services might not have been culturally accessible.
5. **High intelligence or academic success**: Intellectual ability often compensates for autistic challenges, leading to the false assumption that you couldn't be autistic if you succeeded academically.
6. **Supportive early environment**: If your childhood environment accommodated your needs—predictable routines, understanding of sensory needs, acceptance of

interests—you might not have shown enough distress for diagnosis.
7. **Misdiagnosis**: You might have received other diagnoses that partially explained your experiences—anxiety, ADHD, depression—without recognizing underlying autism.
8. **Lack of awareness**: Your parents, teachers, and doctors might simply not have known about autism beyond stereotypes. Autism wasn't widely understood or discussed until recently.

Not being diagnosed in childhood doesn't make your autism less real or valid. Many autistic adults describe diagnosis as solving a lifelong puzzle—suddenly understanding why they've always felt different. Your childhood memories, viewed through an autistic lens, likely contain numerous signs that were misunderstood or dismissed at the time.

Key Takeaways

- Autism diagnostic criteria evolved from narrow definitions focused on young boys to recognizing diverse presentations across genders and ages
- Gender bias in research and clinical practice led to generations of missed diagnoses, particularly among women and gender-diverse individuals
- Cultural factors significantly influence how autism presents and whether it gets recognized, with diagnostic tools showing inherent cultural bias
- The "lost generation" of undiagnosed adults developed complex coping mechanisms while navigating life without understanding their neurological differences
- Autism presentation changes across the lifespan, with adult presentations often looking different from childhood stereotypes

- Multiple intersecting factors—from masking abilities to cultural interpretations—explain why many autistic adults weren't diagnosed as children
- Late diagnosis is increasingly common and valid, offering explanation and self-understanding even decades after childhood

Chapter 3: Adult Autism Presentation

Walking through life feeling like you're operating with a different instruction manual than everyone else—this is how many late-diagnosed autistic adults describe their pre-diagnosis experience. Adult autism presentation often looks radically different from childhood stereotypes, shaped by decades of adaptation, compensation, and survival strategies. Understanding these adult-specific presentations helps explain why so many autistic people remain unrecognized until well into adulthood.

Masking and Camouflaging Behaviors

Masking, also called camouflaging or compensation, refers to the conscious or unconscious suppression of autistic traits to appear more neurotypical (27). Nearly all autistic adults engage in some form of masking, though the intensity and awareness vary considerably. This social survival strategy often begins in early childhood and becomes so automatic that many autistic adults don't realize they're doing it until diagnosis.

Masking encompasses a wide range of behaviors and strategies:

- **Scripting**: Preparing conversational responses in advance, memorizing appropriate reactions
- **Mirroring**: Copying others' body language, facial expressions, and speech patterns
- **Suppressing stims**: Replacing visible stims with subtle ones (leg bouncing instead of rocking)
- **Forcing eye contact**: Despite discomfort or distraction
- **Social studying**: Analyzing social situations like academic subjects
- **Energy management**: Limiting social exposure to maintain the mask

- **Character development**: Creating different "personas" for different situations

Lisa, a 36-year-old human resources manager, describes her masking as "running personality software." She maintains detailed mental files on coworkers—their interests, communication styles, appropriate topics. Before meetings, she reviews her notes and selects which "version" of herself to present. Her work persona laughs at jokes she doesn't understand, makes small talk about topics she finds mundane, and maintains eye contact by looking at people's foreheads. This performance earned her professional success but at tremendous personal cost.

The development of masking often follows predictable patterns. Young autistic children might begin by noticing their differences cause negative reactions. They start suppressing behaviors that draw criticism—hiding their hands to avoid flapping, forcing themselves to play with peers despite preferring solitude. By adolescence, many have developed sophisticated masking strategies, studying popular peers like anthropologists studying foreign cultures.

Michael's masking journey began at age seven when classmates mocked his excitement about cloud formations. He learned to contain his joy, transforming visible happiness into internal pressure. By high school, he'd crafted a "cool guy" persona—hands in pockets (preventing flapping), minimal facial expressions (hiding genuine reactions), strategic silence (avoiding info-dumping). His mask was so effective that when he finally sought autism assessment at 34, his therapist initially dismissed the possibility because he seemed "too socially adept."

The cognitive load of masking is immense. Imagine simultaneously translating a foreign language, solving complex math problems, and performing Shakespeare—all while trying to have a casual conversation. Autistic adults describe the exhaustion of:

- Monitoring their body language constantly
- Translating nonliteral language in real-time
- Suppressing natural responses while calculating appropriate ones
- Managing sensory overload while appearing calm
- Remembering which persona to present to which person

This constant performance has serious consequences. Research links extensive masking to:

- **Autistic burnout**: Complete physical and mental exhaustion
- **Mental health issues**: Depression, anxiety, suicidal ideation
- **Identity confusion**: Losing sense of authentic self
- **Delayed diagnosis**: Masking hides traits from clinicians
- **Physical health problems**: Chronic stress effects
- **Relationship difficulties**: Partners know only the mask

The gender difference in masking is particularly stark. Women and gender-diverse individuals often face stronger social pressure to mask, starting younger and developing more elaborate strategies (28). This contributes to later diagnosis and higher rates of mental health issues among autistic women.

Compensatory Strategies Developed Over Time

Beyond masking social differences, autistic adults develop numerous compensatory strategies to navigate a world designed for neurotypical brains. These strategies often become so integrated that the person doesn't recognize them as autism-related accommodations until diagnosis (29).

Environmental Compensations:

- Choosing careers with minimal social demands or clear interaction rules
- Living alone or with understanding partners who accept autistic needs
- Shopping during off-peak hours to avoid crowds
- Creating detailed organization systems others see as "obsessive"
- Using technology to minimize phone calls and face-to-face interaction

Sarah, a 45-year-old librarian, structured her entire life around unrecognized autistic needs. She chose library science for its quiet environment and rule-based interactions. Her apartment follows strict organizational principles—items grouped by function, then color, then size. She grocery shops at 6 AM on Tuesdays, following the same route through empty aisles. Friends joke about her "quirky routines," never realizing these strategies prevent sensory overload and executive function crashes.

Cognitive Compensations:

- Creating mental flowcharts for social situations
- Developing elaborate planning systems for basic tasks
- Using intelligence to logic through social rules
- Building "decision trees" for common interactions
- Maintaining lists and reminders for everything

Social Compensations:

- Arriving early to avoid entrance anxiety
- Having "escape plans" for all social situations
- Limiting friendships to manageable numbers
- Choosing partners who complement autistic traits
- Creating "social scripts" for different contexts

Sensory Compensations:

- Wearing the same clothing types to avoid texture issues
- Carrying sensory tools disguised as normal items
- Creating sensory-friendly spaces at home and work
- Developing subtle stims that go unnoticed
- Using substances to dull sensory overload

Tom's compensatory strategies evolved over 40 years. As a child, he covered his ears during assemblies. As a teen, he discovered earplugs hidden by long hair. In college, he scheduled classes to avoid peak campus times. As an adult architect, he designed his office with specific lighting, worked with noise-canceling headphones, and specialized in residential projects he could largely complete alone. Each strategy built upon previous ones, creating an elaborate system that supported his success while hiding his autism.

Many compensatory strategies have double edges. The detailed planning that prevents executive function issues can appear as "control freak" behavior. The scripts that enable social interaction prevent genuine connection. The career choices that accommodate autistic needs might not align with interests or abilities. Understanding these as autism-related compensations rather than personality flaws can be profoundly liberating.

Executive Function Challenges in Adult Life

Executive function—the mental processes enabling planning, focus, memory, and multitasking—presents unique challenges for autistic adults. While children might have parents managing executive function demands, adults face these challenges independently in contexts with real consequences (30).

Planning and Prioritization: Autistic adults often struggle with:

- Breaking large tasks into steps
- Estimating time requirements

- Prioritizing competing demands
- Adjusting plans when circumstances change
- Initiating tasks without external structure

Amanda, a talented graphic designer, nearly lost her freelance business before diagnosis. She could create brilliant designs but couldn't manage project timelines, invoice clients, or prioritize assignments. Her desk contained half-finished projects buried under newer ones. She'd hyperfocus on perfecting minor details while missing major deadlines. Post-diagnosis, she hired a virtual assistant for executive function support and created visual project tracking systems that externalized her planning process.

Working Memory and Task Switching: Many autistic adults report:

- Losing track of multi-step processes
- Difficulty resuming interrupted tasks
- Problems juggling multiple responsibilities
- Forgetting daily tasks without reminders
- Struggling with open-ended assignments

Time Blindness: The autistic experience of time often differs from neurotypical expectations:

- Losing hours to hyperfocus
- Underestimating task duration
- Difficulty sensing time passing
- Struggling with scheduling and appointments
- Chronic lateness despite best efforts

Decision Fatigue: The combination of processing differences and sensory sensitivities can make decision-making exhausting:

- Overwhelming options in stores or restaurants
- Analysis paralysis over minor choices

- Difficulty weighing abstract factors
- Needing extensive research before decisions
- Shutdown when faced with too many choices

These executive function challenges intersect with adult responsibilities in complex ways. Managing household tasks, maintaining relationships, advancing careers, and raising children all require executive function skills that don't come naturally to many autistic brains. The gap between intellectual ability and executive function capacity can be particularly frustrating for intellectually gifted autistic adults who excel in their areas of interest but struggle with "simple" daily tasks.

Sensory Differences in Adult Contexts

Sensory processing differences remain a core feature of autism throughout life, but adult contexts present unique sensory challenges. While children might have meltdowns over scratchy clothes or loud noises, adults must navigate sensory issues in professional settings, intimate relationships, and public spaces where accommodations aren't readily available (31).

Workplace Sensory Challenges:

- Open office plans creating constant auditory intrusion
- Fluorescent lighting causing headaches and disorientation
- Perfumes and cleaning products triggering nausea
- Business clothing textures causing physical distress
- Temperature variations affecting concentration

Robert, a software engineer, spent years battling invisible sensory assaults at work. The air conditioning's hum made thinking feel like swimming through mud. His coworker's keyboard clicking sent sharp pains through his skull. The required business casual clothes felt like sandpaper. He developed chronic migraines, attributed to "stress," before recognizing them as sensory overload. Post-diagnosis, he negotiated remote work and transformed his home office into a sensory sanctuary.

Social Setting Sensory Issues:

- Restaurant noise preventing conversation tracking
- Party environments causing complete overload
- Physical touch expectations in social contexts
- Competing sensory input in group settings
- Alcohol use to dull sensory overwhelm

Intimate Relationship Sensory Factors:

- Touch sensitivity affecting physical intimacy
- Sound sensitivity to breathing or movement
- Need for specific pressure or texture
- Difficulty with spontaneous physical contact
- Mismatched sensory needs between partners

Daily Life Sensory Management: Adult autistic people develop numerous strategies for sensory regulation:

- Carrying "survival kits" with sensory tools
- Planning routes to avoid sensory triggers
- Creating detailed routines minimizing sensory stress
- Using technology for sensory accommodation
- Building recovery time into schedules

The cumulative effect of daily sensory assaults contributes significantly to autistic burnout. Unlike children who might have parents advocating for sensory accommodations, adults must self-advocate in environments where sensory needs are often dismissed as "preferences" or "being difficult."

Social Communication in Professional Settings

Professional environments present unique social communication challenges for autistic adults. The unwritten rules of workplace interaction, office politics, and professional networking can feel like navigating a minefield without a map (32). Many autistic adults develop elaborate strategies for managing professional communication, though these often come at significant personal cost.

Meeting Dynamics: Professional meetings combine multiple challenging elements:

- Rapid topic switching requiring mental flexibility
- Nonverbal cues indicating speaking turns
- Expected small talk before/after business
- Group dynamics and power hierarchies
- Pressure for immediate verbal responses

Jennifer, a project manager at a tech company, spent her first decade developing meeting survival strategies. She arrives ten minutes early to claim a seat with wall support and clear sightlines. She brings detailed agendas with scripted contributions. She's learned to count to three before speaking to avoid interrupting and practices active listening poses while processing information. Her "meeting persona" appears engaged and collaborative, but she schedules nothing afterward, knowing she'll need recovery time.

Networking Challenges: Professional networking epitomizes everything difficult about neurotypical social interaction:

- Surface-level conversation about multiple topics
- Remembering names and faces in overwhelming environments
- Managing sensory overload while appearing professional
- Understanding hidden agendas and ulterior motives
- Following up appropriately without seeming pushy

Email and Digital Communication: While many autistic adults prefer written communication, professional email has its own challenges:

- Interpreting tone in written messages
- Understanding implied vs. stated requests
- Managing the anxiety of unclear expectations
- Crafting appropriately "warm" professional tone
- Knowing when to escalate from email to phone

Workplace Social Expectations: Beyond formal communication, workplaces have numerous unwritten social rules:

- Participating in casual "water cooler" conversation
- Attending optional social events
- Understanding office humor and sarcasm
- Managing workplace friendships appropriately
- Navigating office politics and alliances

David's experience illustrates these challenges. As a financial analyst, his numerical skills earned recognition, but social expectations nearly derailed his career. He couldn't understand why colleagues discussed weekends when there was work to do. He answered "How are you?" honestly, describing his chronic insomnia and sensory overload. He missed "optional" happy hours, not realizing they were politically mandatory. His direct communication style, while efficient, was labeled "abrasive." Only after diagnosis did he understand these weren't personal failings but autism-related communication differences.

Many autistic adults find success in fields with clearer communication rules or minimal social demands. Others develop extensive masking strategies for professional settings, maintaining a "work self" entirely separate from their authentic identity. The energy required for this constant translation between autistic and neurotypical communication styles contributes significantly to professional burnout.

FAQ: "How do I know if I'm masking?"

Recognizing masking can be challenging because it often becomes so automatic you don't realize you're doing it. Here are signs you might be masking:

During Social Interactions:

- You rehearse conversations beforehand, even casual ones
- You consciously monitor your body language and facial expressions
- You suppress natural reactions (stimming, honest responses)
- You feel like you're "performing" rather than being yourself
- You copy others' expressions and mannerisms
- You force eye contact despite discomfort

After Social Interactions:

- You feel exhausted, even from "successful" socializing
- You need alone time to "recharge" more than seems typical
- You replay conversations, analyzing what you did wrong
- You experience delayed emotional reactions
- You have physical symptoms (headaches, muscle tension)

Long-term Patterns:

- Different people know completely different versions of you
- You've been called "fake" when you thought you were being polite

- You struggle to identify your own preferences and needs
- You feel like you're constantly failing despite trying so hard
- You've lost touch with who you really are
- You experience cycles of burnout from maintaining the mask

Unmasking Signs: Conversely, you might notice masking by how different you feel when not masking:

- With certain safe people, you're completely different
- Alone, you engage in behaviors you hide from others
- You have specific places where you can "be yourself"
- Vacation or stress brings out your "real" self
- You notice huge relief when you can drop the act

Masking isn't inherently bad—it's a survival strategy in a neurotypical world. However, recognizing when and how you mask helps you make conscious choices about when it's necessary versus when you can be more authentic. Many late-diagnosed adults describe diagnosis as permission to unmask, at least partially, leading to better mental health and self-acceptance.

Key Takeaways

- Masking involves consciously or unconsciously suppressing autistic traits to appear neurotypical, often at significant personal cost
- Adult autistic people develop elaborate compensatory strategies across all life areas, from career choices to living arrangements
- Executive function challenges in planning, time management, and task switching create unique difficulties in adult responsibilities

- Sensory processing differences persist throughout life but manifest differently in adult contexts like workplaces and relationships
- Professional environments require complex social communication skills that many autistic adults find exhausting to navigate
- Recognizing masking and compensatory strategies is often the first step toward self-understanding and seeking diagnosis
- The cumulative effect of masking, compensation, and managing daily challenges contributes to autistic burnout and mental health issues

Understanding how autism presents in adulthood opens the door to recognition and, ultimately, diagnosis. The patterns discussed—masking, compensation, executive function challenges, sensory differences, and social communication struggles—form a constellation that many adults suddenly recognize as their lifelong experience. The next chapter explores how to transform this recognition into formal diagnosis, navigating the complex landscape of adult autism assessment and the emotional journey it entails.

Chapter 4: Self-Discovery and Pre-Diagnosis

That moment of recognition can arrive unexpectedly—scrolling through social media, reading an article, watching a video where someone describes their autistic experience, and suddenly your entire life makes sense. For many adults, the path to autism diagnosis begins not in a doctor's office but in quiet moments of self-discovery, often accompanied by equal measures of relief and disbelief. This chapter guides you through the self-identification process, from those first inklings of recognition through preparing for formal assessment.

Common Paths to Self-Identification

The routes to recognizing autism in yourself rarely follow straight lines. Most adults who seek diagnosis later in life describe a gradual accumulation of clues rather than a single revelatory moment. Understanding these common pathways can help validate your own journey and provide a framework for organizing your experiences.

Through Your Children Perhaps the most common path to adult diagnosis begins in pediatric waiting rooms. Parents attending their child's autism assessment often experience profound recognition as clinicians describe traits they've managed their entire lives.

Sandra, a 38-year-old accountant, accompanied her daughter Maya to an autism evaluation. As the psychologist explained how autistic girls might organize their toys by color rather than playing imaginatively, Sandra flashed back to her own childhood bedroom—stuffed animals arranged in rainbow order, dolls lined up by height. When the clinician discussed masking behaviors, Sandra realized she'd been teaching Maya her own coping strategies without recognizing them as such. "I thought I was helping her be 'normal,'" Sandra recalls. "Then I understood we were both autistic, just very good at hiding it."

Through Mental Health Treatment Many adults discover autism while seeking help for anxiety, depression, or other mental health concerns. Therapists trained in recognizing autism may notice patterns that previous providers missed.

Marcus spent fifteen years in therapy for treatment-resistant depression. His sixth therapist, reviewing his history, noticed something others had overlooked. His depression worsened after social events. His anxiety peaked in environments with fluorescent lighting. His "rigid thinking" that previous therapists tried to fix actually helped him excel as a computer programmer. When she suggested autism screening, Marcus initially dismissed it—he had friends, a job, a degree. But the screening results led to comprehensive assessment and, finally, accurate diagnosis at age 34.

Through Online Communities Social media and online forums have revolutionized autism self-discovery. Autistic adults sharing their experiences create recognition cascades as others see themselves reflected in these narratives.

Elena discovered autism through TikTok, of all places. The algorithm, noting her interest in ADHD content, began showing her videos by autistic creators. One video about "weird things that are actually autism" included her exact bedtime routine— the same audiobook every night, blankets arranged in specific order, white noise at precise volume. She fell down what she calls "the autism rabbit hole," consuming content that explained everything from her texture-based eating to her inability to maintain friendships. Six months later, she pursued formal diagnosis.

Through Relationship Patterns Some adults recognize autism through repeated relationship difficulties that finally form a pattern. Partners, friends, or family members might also suggest the possibility.

James had three failed marriages before age 45. Each wife complained about the same issues—his need for routine, his literal interpretation of language, his meltdowns when plans changed, his "emotional distance." His fourth partner, who worked in special education, gently suggested he might be autistic. Initially offended, James began researching, finding his entire relationship history reframed through an autism lens. "I wasn't a bad husband," he reflects. "I was an undiagnosed autistic husband trying to navigate neurotypical expectations without a map."

Through Career Challenges Workplace difficulties, especially around communication and sensory issues, can trigger autism recognition. This particularly affects adults who excelled academically but struggle professionally.

Dr. Chen breezed through medical school and residency, her exceptional memory and pattern recognition making her an outstanding diagnostician. But as an attending physician, she struggled. Small talk with colleagues exhausted her. The hospital's constant noise and bright lights triggered daily headaches. She couldn't understand workplace politics, inadvertently offending administrators with her direct communication. When a colleague mentioned her own autism diagnosis, Dr. Chen saw herself clearly for the first time.

Online Assessments and Screening Tools

The internet offers numerous autism screening tools, varying widely in quality and purpose. Understanding how to use these tools appropriately—and their limitations—helps make self-discovery more structured and prepares you for professional assessment.

Validated Screening Tools Available Online:

The **Autism Spectrum Quotient (AQ)** remains the most widely used screening tool. Developed by Simon Baron-Cohen and colleagues, this 50-question assessment measures autistic traits across five domains: social skills, attention switching, attention to detail, communication, and imagination (33). Scores above 32 suggest significant autistic traits, though cultural factors affect scoring.

The **Camouflaging Autistic Traits Questionnaire (CAT-Q)** specifically measures masking behaviors, particularly useful for adults who've developed strong compensatory strategies (34). High CAT-Q scores might explain why other screening tools miss your autism.

The **Ritvo Autism Asperger Diagnostic Scale-Revised (RAADS-R)** includes 80 questions examining developmental and current symptoms (35). Its strength lies in distinguishing autism from other conditions, though its length can be overwhelming.

Using Screening Tools Effectively:

- Take multiple assessments for a fuller picture
- Complete them when you're rested and can focus
- Answer based on your internal experience, not how you appear to others
- Consider both current traits and childhood experiences
- Save your results for sharing with diagnosticians

Sarah's screening journey illustrates effective tool use. She started with the AQ, scoring 28—below the typical threshold. Frustrated but still recognizing herself in autism descriptions, she took the CAT-Q, discovering extremely high masking scores. The RAADS-R revealed significant autism traits hidden by her compensatory strategies. Armed with these results, she felt confident pursuing professional assessment.

Limitations to Understand:

- Screening tools aren't diagnostic—they indicate whether assessment might be worthwhile
- Cultural bias affects all current tools
- High masking can lead to false negatives
- Other conditions (anxiety, ADHD, trauma) can inflate scores
- No tool captures the full autism experience

Building Your Case History

Creating a comprehensive personal history strengthens your self-understanding and provides valuable information for professional assessment. This process involves systematic documentation of traits, experiences, and patterns throughout your life.

Organizing Current Experiences:

Start with present-day experiences, as these are freshest in memory. Document:

- **Sensory experiences**: Which lights, sounds, textures, or smells cause distress? What sensory input do you seek for comfort?
- **Communication patterns**: Do you interpret language literally? Struggle with subtext? Script conversations?
- **Social experiences**: How do social interactions affect you? What strategies do you use?
- **Executive function**: Document planning difficulties, time blindness, task-switching challenges
- **Special interests**: Current and past intense interests, including duration and depth

- **Routines and rituals**: Daily patterns that provide structure and comfort
- **Meltdowns/shutdowns**: Triggers, warning signs, recovery needs

Maria created a spreadsheet tracking daily experiences for three months. She noted energy levels before and after social interactions, sensory triggers throughout each day, and communication challenges. Patterns emerged—Mondays were hardest due to fluorescent office lighting, video calls drained her more than in-person meetings, and she needed exactly 45 minutes of silence after work before she could speak comfortably.

Gathering Historical Evidence:

Childhood evidence strengthens adult diagnosis, though gaps in memory are normal. Gather:

- School reports mentioning behavioral observations
- Photos showing repetitive play, unusual interests, or sensory behaviors
- Medical records noting developmental differences
- Family stories about your quirks or challenges
- Creative writing revealing literal thinking or special interests
- Report cards with teacher comments

Creating Trait Timelines:

Develop chronological timelines showing how traits manifested across life stages:

Age 5-10: Lined up toys, echolalia, read encyclopedia for fun, no friends *Age 11-15:* Developed first special interest (astronomy), learned to force eye contact, daily meltdowns at home *Age 16-20:* Studied popular kids to learn social rules, developed eating disorder, excelled academically *Age 21-30:* Chose career minimizing social interaction, first autistic burnout, relationship difficulties *Age 31-present:* Chronic anxiety/depression, sensory issues worsening, seeking answers

Documenting Childhood Experiences

Childhood documentation presents unique challenges for adult diagnosis. Many adults lack access to early records, have unreliable family narratives, or experienced trauma that complicates memory retrieval. Strategic approaches help maximize available evidence.

Interview Strategies for Family Members:

When interviewing family about your childhood, avoid mentioning autism initially. Instead, ask open-ended questions:

- "What was I like as a small child?"
- "Did I have any unusual habits or interests?"
- "How did I play differently from other children?"
- "What did teachers say about me?"
- "What family stories exist about my quirks?"

Thomas discovered crucial information through strategic family interviews. His mother, initially dismissive of autism possibility, shared extensive stories when asked generally about his childhood. She described how he organized Halloween candy by wrapper color before eating, insisted on wearing the same outfit daily in second grade, and taught himself to read at three but couldn't tie shoes until age ten. These concrete examples proved invaluable during assessment.

Alternative Evidence Sources:

When family history isn't available or reliable, consider:

- **Home videos or audio recordings**: Look for stimming, echolalia, unusual play
- **School yearbooks**: Often contain candid behavioral observations
- **Childhood creations**: Drawings, stories, or projects revealing special interests
- **Medical records**: Even unrelated visits might note behavioral observations
- **Siblings or childhood friends**: May recall details parents normalized

Addressing Memory Gaps:

Trauma, dissociation, and time can create significant memory gaps. Address these by:

- Focusing on sensory memories, which often remain vivid
- Using photos or objects to trigger recollections
- Accepting partial memories as valid evidence
- Documenting what you can't remember as potentially trauma-related
- Recognizing that memory gaps themselves might indicate childhood distress

Preparing for Professional Assessment

Thorough preparation maximizes the value of professional assessment while reducing anxiety about the process. Understanding what assessors need and organizing your information systematically creates better outcomes.

Creating Assessment Documentation:

Organize your self-discovery materials into a comprehensive packet:

1. **Executive Summary**: One-page overview of why you're seeking assessment
2. **Screening Results**: All completed assessments with dates and scores
3. **Trait Examples**: Specific, concrete examples organized by DSM-5 criteria
4. **Historical Timeline**: Life history showing trait development
5. **Impact Statement**: How traits affect daily functioning
6. **Previous Diagnoses**: Mental health history and treatments
7. **Questions List**: What you hope to learn from assessment

Lisa's preparation packet impressed her diagnostician. Her executive summary clearly stated: "Seeking autism assessment after recognizing lifelong patterns following daughter's diagnosis. Significant masking makes traits less obvious but profoundly impacts daily functioning." She organized fifty pages of documentation with tabs, making information easily accessible during the assessment.

Practical Preparation Steps:

- **Research your assessor**: Understand their methods and autism knowledge
- **Practice discussing difficulties**: Many autistic adults minimize struggles
- **Prepare sensory accommodations**: Request environmental modifications
- **Plan recovery time**: Schedule nothing after assessment
- **Consider support person**: Some assessors allow advocates present
- **Document current medications**: Some affect assessment results

Managing Pre-Assessment Anxiety:

Assessment anxiety is nearly universal. Address it by:

- Recognizing that assessment is collaborative exploration, not testing
- Understanding that "failing" assessment doesn't invalidate your experiences
- Preparing scripts for difficult topics
- Planning comfort items or stims for the appointment
- Knowing you can take breaks if needed
- Accepting that showing authentic struggles helps accurate diagnosis

Chapter FAQ: "Should I self-diagnose?"

Self-diagnosis in the autistic community is widely accepted and valid for many reasons. Professional diagnosis isn't accessible to everyone due to cost, availability, cultural barriers, or discrimination risk. Many autistic adults find self-diagnosis sufficient for understanding themselves and accessing community support.

Valid reasons for self-diagnosis:

- **Financial barriers**: Assessment costs thousands of dollars
- **Geographic limitations**: No qualified assessors nearby
- **Long waitlists**: Often 1-2 years for adult assessment
- **Discrimination concerns**: Formal diagnosis can affect custody, immigration, insurance
- **Cultural barriers**: Assessment tools aren't culturally adapted
- **Previous misdiagnosis**: Past psychiatric treatment creating provider bias

Benefits of self-diagnosis:

- Immediate access to community support and resources

- Framework for understanding your experiences
- Permission to implement accommodations
- Identity validation without external gatekeeping
- Avoiding potentially traumatic assessment experiences

When to seek formal diagnosis:

- Needing workplace or educational accommodations
- Accessing disability benefits or services
- Wanting professional validation
- Ruling out other conditions
- Personal closure or family acceptance

The self-diagnosis versus formal diagnosis decision is deeply personal. Many self-diagnosed autistic adults contribute meaningfully to the community and live fulfilling lives without professional validation. Others find formal diagnosis necessary for practical or emotional reasons. Both paths are valid.

David self-diagnosed at 42 after extensive research. He joined online autistic communities, implemented sensory accommodations, and finally understood his lifelong struggles. Two years later, needing workplace accommodations, he pursued formal assessment. The psychologist confirmed what David already knew, but having documentation enabled him to request the support he needed while maintaining the self-knowledge that preceded professional validation.

Key Takeaways

- Multiple pathways lead to autism self-identification, including through children's diagnoses, mental health treatment, online communities, relationship patterns, and workplace challenges
- Online screening tools provide structured self-assessment but have limitations including cultural bias and masking effects

- Building a comprehensive case history requires documenting current experiences, gathering childhood evidence, and creating trait timelines
- Childhood documentation can come from many sources beyond memory, including family interviews, school records, and creative artifacts
- Preparing thoroughly for assessment includes organizing documentation, managing anxiety, and understanding the process
- Self-diagnosis is valid and accepted within the autistic community, with formal diagnosis being one option among many
- The self-discovery process itself provides valuable self-understanding regardless of ultimate diagnosis decisions

Self-discovery often marks the beginning rather than end of the autism journey. You've recognized patterns, documented experiences, and prepared for whatever comes next. The following chapter explores the formal diagnosis process—finding qualified professionals, understanding assessment types, and managing the practical aspects of seeking professional validation. For those choosing formal assessment, your self-discovery work provides the foundation for meaningful diagnostic exploration.

Chapter 5: Getting a Professional Diagnosis

The decision to pursue formal autism diagnosis as an adult often comes after months or years of self-reflection, research, and internal debate. Once you've decided to seek assessment, you face a new set of challenges—finding qualified professionals, understanding assessment options, managing costs, and navigating systems designed primarily for children. This chapter provides a practical roadmap through the professional diagnosis process, helping you make informed decisions at each step.

Finding Qualified Diagnosticians

Locating professionals qualified to diagnose autism in adults presents the first major hurdle. Many clinicians experienced with childhood autism lack training in adult presentation, particularly in recognizing masked traits. Understanding the types of professionals who can diagnose and how to evaluate their qualifications saves time, money, and potential misdiagnosis heartache.

Who Can Diagnose Autism:

Different professionals have diagnostic capabilities, varying by location and healthcare system:

- **Psychologists**: Often most experienced with autism assessment, particularly neuropsychologists and clinical psychologists specializing in developmental conditions
- **Psychiatrists**: Medical doctors who can diagnose and prescribe medication if needed for co-occurring conditions
- **Neurologists**: Sometimes involved in autism diagnosis, particularly when ruling out other neurological conditions

- **Developmental Pediatricians**: Occasionally see adults, especially young adults transitioning from pediatric care
- **Multidisciplinary Teams**: Some centers use teams combining various specialists

Evaluating Diagnostician Qualifications:

Not all licensed professionals understand adult autism presentation. Ask potential diagnosticians:

1. How many adult autism assessments have you conducted?
2. What training have you received specifically on adult autism?
3. How do you account for masking and camouflaging in assessment?
4. What's your understanding of autism presentation differences across genders?
5. Which assessment tools do you use for adults?
6. What's your perspective on self-diagnosis and late diagnosis?

Rachel's search illustrates the importance of vetting providers. Her first psychologist dismissed her concerns, saying, "You made eye contact and have a job—you can't be autistic." The second relied entirely on childhood-focused questionnaires. Finally, she found Dr. Martinez, who specialized in adult autism and understood how decades of masking could hide traits. The difference in assessment quality was profound.

Red Flags to Avoid:

- Professionals who believe autism is only a childhood condition
- Those using only childhood-focused assessment tools
- Clinicians who dismiss self-diagnosis research entirely
- Providers who claim you "don't look autistic"

- Anyone guaranteeing diagnosis (or non-diagnosis) before assessment
- Professionals unfamiliar with current DSM-5 criteria

Finding Specialists:

Search strategies for qualified diagnosticians:

- **Professional directories**: Psychology Today allows filtering by specialty
- **Autism organizations**: Local and national organizations maintain referral lists
- **Adult autism clinics**: Specialized centers in major cities or universities
- **Online communities**: Other late-diagnosed adults share recommendations
- **Telehealth options**: Expands access to qualified specialists
- **Medical schools**: University-affiliated clinics often have specialists

Types of Assessments Available

Adult autism assessments vary significantly in depth, duration, and approach. Understanding different assessment types helps you choose appropriately based on your needs, resources, and diagnostic complexity.

Comprehensive Neuropsychological Assessment:

The gold standard involves extensive testing across multiple domains:

- **Clinical interviews**: Detailed developmental history and current functioning
- **Cognitive testing**: IQ assessment, executive function, processing speed

- **Autism-specific measures**: ADOS-2, ADI-R, specialist questionnaires
- **Psychological testing**: Personality assessment, mental health screening
- **Adaptive functioning**: Daily living skills evaluation
- **Sensory assessment**: Formal sensory profile evaluation

Duration: 6-20 hours across multiple sessions Cost: $3,000-$6,000 Best for: Complex cases, co-occurring conditions, thorough documentation needs

Focused Autism Assessment:

Streamlined evaluation targeting autism specifically:

- **Structured clinical interview**: Based on DSM-5 criteria
- **Autism screening tools**: Multiple validated questionnaires
- **Behavioral observation**: May include modified ADOS-2
- **Developmental history**: Focus on autism-relevant experiences
- **Functional impact assessment**: Current life effects

Duration: 2-6 hours, often single session Cost: $800-$2,500 Best for: Clear autism presentation, limited co-occurring conditions

Psychiatric Diagnostic Evaluation:

Psychiatrist-conducted assessment:

- **Clinical interview**: Mental health and developmental history
- **Diagnostic screening**: Broad mental health assessment
- **Medication evaluation**: If relevant for co-occurring conditions
- **DSM-5 criteria review**: Systematic autism evaluation

Duration: 1-3 hours Cost: $500-$1,500 Best for: Those needing medication management, insurance coverage

Michael's assessment journey shows how choice matters. Initially, he pursued comprehensive neuropsychological testing, spending $4,500 and enduring 15 hours of testing. The extensive cognitive testing felt irrelevant to his autism questions. His partner, seeking diagnosis later, chose focused autism assessment with a specialist, receiving equally valid diagnosis in 4 hours for $1,200.

What to Expect During Evaluation

Understanding the assessment process reduces anxiety and improves preparation. While specific procedures vary by clinician and assessment type, common elements exist across most adult evaluations.

Pre-Assessment Phase:

Before meeting, expect:

- Extensive intake paperwork about development and current functioning
- Requests for childhood records or informant participation
- Screening questionnaires to complete at home
- Insurance verification and payment arrangements
- Consent forms explaining the assessment process

Clinical Interview Component:

The interview forms assessment's core, typically covering:

- **Developmental history**: Early milestones, childhood behaviors, school experiences

- **Social communication**: Friendship patterns, relationship history, communication challenges
- **Restricted/repetitive behaviors**: Special interests, routines, sensory experiences
- **Current functioning**: Work, relationships, daily living impacts
- **Mental health history**: Previous diagnoses, treatments, trauma
- **Family history**: Neurodevelopmental conditions in relatives

Jennifer's interview experience highlights thorough assessment. Her psychologist spent three hours exploring her life history, asking detailed questions about childhood play patterns, teenage social experiences, and adult coping strategies. The clinician noted not just what Jennifer said but how she said it—her formal language, minimal gesture use, and tendency to provide excessive detail about special interests.

Observational Components:

Clinicians observe various behaviors during assessment:

- Eye contact patterns and quality
- Gesture use and body language
- Conversational turn-taking
- Response to topic changes
- Emotional expression range
- Stimming or self-soothing behaviors
- Reaction to sensory stimuli in the office

Structured Activities (if using ADOS-2):

Some assessments include structured interactions:

- Telling stories from pictures
- Describing abstract images

- Demonstrating tasks
- Conversational exercises
- Joint attention activities
- Play-based scenarios (adapted for adults)

Cognitive or Additional Testing:

Depending on assessment type:

- IQ testing to establish cognitive profile
- Executive function assessment
- Attention and memory testing
- Academic achievement screening
- Personality assessment
- Trauma screening

Post-Assessment Process:

After evaluation sessions:

- Clinician scores and interprets all data
- Report writing (2-4 weeks typical)
- Feedback session to discuss results
- Written report provided
- Recommendations for support
- Referrals if needed

Cost Considerations and Insurance

The financial burden of adult autism assessment creates significant access barriers. Understanding costs, insurance possibilities, and alternative funding helps make assessment more attainable.

Typical Cost Ranges:

Assessment costs vary by type, location, and provider:

- **Major cities**: $2,000-$6,000 for comprehensive assessment
- **Suburban areas**: $1,500-$4,000 typically
- **Rural areas**: May be lower but require travel costs
- **Telehealth**: Sometimes lower overhead reduces costs
- **University clinics**: Often offer sliding scales
- **Private practice**: Generally most expensive

Insurance Coverage Challenges:

Insurance coverage for adult autism assessment remains inconsistent:

- Many insurers consider adult assessment "not medically necessary"
- Some require prior authorization with extensive documentation
- Coverage may depend on billing codes used
- Mental health benefits may have different coverage than medical
- Out-of-network providers require reimbursement navigation

David's insurance battle illustrates common challenges. His insurer initially denied coverage, claiming autism assessment wasn't necessary for adults. After three appeals, providing research on adult diagnosis importance, and getting his primary care physician involved, he received partial coverage. The process took four months but saved $2,000.

Strategies for Managing Costs:

- **Payment plans**: Many providers offer extended payment options
- **FSA/HSA funds**: Use pre-tax healthcare dollars
- **Sliding scale options**: Ask about income-based fees

- **University training clinics**: Supervised students offer reduced rates
- **Grant programs**: Some organizations offer diagnostic scholarships
- **Employer assistance programs**: EAPs sometimes cover assessment
- **Crowd-funding**: Community support for diagnosis costs

Documentation for Insurance:

When seeking reimbursement:

1. Get detailed receipts with procedure codes
2. Request a "superbill" for out-of-network claims
3. Obtain letter of medical necessity from referring provider
4. Document all communications with insurance
5. Appeal denials with supporting research
6. Consider involving patient advocates

International Differences in Diagnostic Processes

Autism diagnosis procedures vary dramatically worldwide, reflecting different healthcare systems, cultural attitudes, and resource availability. Understanding these differences helps those seeking diagnosis outside their home country or immigrating after diagnosis.

United States:

- Private healthcare dominates adult assessment
- No centralized diagnostic pathway
- Significant state-by-state variations
- Long waitlists in public systems
- High out-of-pocket costs common

United Kingdom:

- NHS provides free assessment but with 2+ year waits
- Right to Choose allows some private provider selection
- Private assessment available for those who can pay
- NICE guidelines standardize assessment approaches
- GP referral typically required

Canada:

- Provincial healthcare coverage varies widely
- Some provinces cover adult assessment, others don't
- Private assessment often necessary
- Significant urban/rural disparities
- French-language assessment availability in Quebec

Australia:

- Medicare provides some rebates for assessment
- Psychiatrist diagnosis required for funding access
- National Disability Insurance Scheme considers autism
- Private assessment common due to public waitlists
- Telehealth increasingly available

European Union:

- Massive country-by-country variation
- Some countries have excellent public provision
- Others lack adult autism services entirely
- Language barriers for expatriates
- EU citizenship may not guarantee access

Amara's international journey demonstrates complexity. Diagnosed in Germany through public healthcare, she moved to the United States for work. Her German diagnosis wasn't automatically accepted. She needed new assessment for workplace accommodations, navigating insurance systems she didn't understand in her second language. The cultural differences in how autism was perceived added another layer of challenge.

Key International Considerations:

- **Diagnosis portability**: Not all countries accept others' diagnoses
- **Language barriers**: Assessment in non-native language affects results
- **Cultural bias**: Assessment tools reflect cultural assumptions
- **Legal implications**: Diagnosis affects immigration in some countries
- **Access variations**: Rural areas globally lack specialists

Chapter FAQ: "How much does diagnosis cost?"

The cost of adult autism diagnosis varies enormously based on multiple factors. Here's a realistic breakdown:

Direct Assessment Costs:

- **Low end**: $500-$1,000 for basic psychiatric evaluation
- **Mid-range**: $1,500-$3,000 for focused autism assessment
- **High end**: $3,000-$6,000+ for comprehensive neuropsychological evaluation

Additional Potential Costs:

- **Travel expenses**: If specialists aren't local
- **Lost wages**: Time off work for assessment
- **Record gathering**: Obtaining childhood documentation
- **Pre-assessment therapy**: Some require referring provider
- **Follow-up services**: Post-diagnosis support

Insurance Coverage Reality: While some insurance plans cover assessment, many adults pay partially or fully out-of-pocket. Coverage depends on:

- Your specific plan benefits
- Whether provider is in-network
- How assessment is coded
- Your persistence in appeals
- State insurance mandates

Budget Planning Suggestions:

1. **Research costs upfront**: Get written estimates
2. **Compare providers**: Prices vary significantly
3. **Ask about payment options**: Many offer plans
4. **Consider timing**: Use FSA/HSA funds strategically
5. **Explore alternatives**: University clinics, telehealth
6. **Factor hidden costs**: Travel, time off, documentation

Cost-Benefit Analysis: Consider diagnosis value against cost:

- Need for workplace accommodations
- Access to support services
- Personal validation importance
- Relationship or family dynamics
- Mental health treatment planning
- Long-term life planning needs

Many adults find diagnosis worthwhile despite high costs. Others decide self-diagnosis suffices given financial barriers. Both decisions are valid. If you need diagnosis but can't afford it, explore every alternative funding option—grants, sliding scales, payment plans, crowd-funding. The autistic community often helps members access diagnosis through resource sharing and financial support.

Key Takeaways

- Finding qualified diagnosticians requires careful vetting, as many professionals lack adult autism expertise
- Assessment types range from comprehensive neuropsychological evaluation to focused autism assessment, each with different costs and benefits
- The evaluation process typically includes clinical interviews, behavioral observation, and potentially structured activities or cognitive testing
- Costs vary dramatically ($500-$6,000+) with limited insurance coverage, requiring strategic financial planning
- International diagnostic processes differ significantly, affecting access and portability of diagnosis
- Multiple funding strategies exist for managing assessment costs, from payment plans to grants
- The decision to pursue formal diagnosis depends on individual needs, resources, and circumstances

Crossing the Threshold

Completing professional assessment marks a significant milestone, regardless of outcome. You've navigated complex systems, invested considerable resources, and opened yourself to clinical scrutiny. The next chapter explores what comes after—processing your diagnosis emotionally, reconstructing identity, managing imposter syndrome, and building support systems. For those receiving autism diagnosis, a new phase of understanding and self-acceptance begins.

Chapter 6: After Your Diagnosis

The email arrives on an ordinary Tuesday, or perhaps you're sitting across from your diagnostician as they say the words: "You meet the criteria for autism spectrum disorder." Time seems to pause. Years of questioning, confusion, and self-doubt crystallize into this moment of validation. Yet diagnosis isn't an ending—it's the beginning of a profound journey of self-discovery, identity reconstruction, and practical life changes. This chapter guides you through the complex landscape that follows diagnosis.

Processing the Diagnosis Emotionally

Receiving an autism diagnosis in adulthood unleashes a cascade of emotions that can feel overwhelming and contradictory. Understanding these emotional responses as normal parts of the diagnostic journey helps you navigate them with self-compassion.

The Initial Response Spectrum:

Adults describe vastly different immediate reactions to diagnosis:

- **Relief**: "Finally, an explanation that makes sense"
- **Validation**: "I'm not broken, lazy, or deliberately difficult"
- **Grief**: "Mourning the support I never received"
- **Anger**: "Why did no one notice? How different could life have been?"
- **Fear**: "What does this mean for my future?"
- **Numbness**: "I need time to process this"
- **Joy**: "I understand myself for the first time"

Katherine, diagnosed at 43, experienced what she calls "emotional whiplash." The first day brought euphoric relief—finally understanding why she'd always felt like an alien attempting to pass as human. Day two brought crushing grief for her younger self who struggled without support. By week's end, anger surfaced about teachers who labeled her "problem child" instead of recognizing her needs. These shifting emotions continued for months.

The Grief Process:

Many adults experience genuine grief following diagnosis, mourning:

- The childhood support they didn't receive
- Relationships lost to misunderstandings
- Career paths derailed by unrecognized struggles
- Years spent believing they were failures
- Energy wasted on unsustainable masking
- Opportunities missed due to lack of accommodations

This grief is valid and necessary. You're mourning alternate life paths that proper support might have enabled. Allow yourself to feel this loss without minimizing it.

Processing Trauma:

Late diagnosis often means decades of trauma from living in a world not designed for your neurology:

- Bullying for being "weird" or "different"
- Punishment for autistic behaviors
- Forced compliance with neurotypical standards
- Gaslighting about your experiences
- Mental health misdiagnoses and inappropriate treatments
- Relationship trauma from communication differences

Marcus realized his diagnosis explained not just his present struggles but past traumas. Teachers punishing him for "defiance" when he needed explicit instructions. Parents forcing eye contact that felt physically painful. Therapists treating his special interests as obsessions requiring extinction. Understanding these as responses to unrecognized autism, not personal failings, began his healing process.

Managing Emotional Intensity:

The post-diagnosis period often intensifies emotions:

1. **Create processing space**: Schedule time for emotional exploration
2. **Use familiar regulation strategies**: Engage special interests, preferred stims
3. **Seek autism-affirming therapy**: Process with someone who understands
4. **Connect with others diagnosed as adults**: Shared experience helps
5. **Document your journey**: Writing or art can aid processing
6. **Be patient with yourself**: Emotional integration takes time

Identity Reconstruction

Autism diagnosis in adulthood necessitates fundamental identity reconstruction. You're not becoming someone new—you're understanding who you've always been through an accurate lens. This process of reframing your entire life through an autistic perspective can be simultaneously liberating and destabilizing.

Rewriting Your Life Story:

Post-diagnosis, many adults engage in comprehensive life review, reinterpreting experiences through an autism framework:

- Childhood "shyness" becomes social communication differences
- Being "picky" reveals sensory processing needs
- "Obsessions" transform into special interests
- "Laziness" is recognized as executive dysfunction
- "Sensitivity" reflects nervous system differences
- "Difficult" behavior was actually autistic distress

Sarah spent months after diagnosis creating what she called her "autism autobiography." She reviewed old photos, report cards, and journals, identifying previously unrecognized autistic traits. Her kindergarten teacher's note about her "unusual attachment to routine" took new meaning. Her teenage diary entries about feeling "like an anthropologist studying humans" suddenly made sense. This reframing felt like solving a lifelong puzzle.

Integrating Autistic Identity:

Identity integration involves several stages:

1. Discovery Phase: Learning about autism beyond stereotypes

- Reading autistic authors, not just clinical texts
- Exploring neurodiversity perspectives
- Understanding autism as neurological difference
- Recognizing internalized ableism

2. Experimentation Phase: Trying new ways of being

- Reducing masking in safe situations
- Acknowledging sensory needs publicly
- Using accommodations without shame
- Expressing authentic communication styles

3. Integration Phase: Developing coherent identity

- Balancing disclosure decisions

- Finding sustainable masking levels
- Advocating for needs appropriately
- Building on autistic strengths

Navigating Multiple Identities:

Autism intersects with all other aspects of identity:

- **Cultural identity**: How autism manifests within cultural contexts
- **Gender identity**: High correlation between autism and gender diversity
- **Sexual orientation**: Increased LGBTQ+ identification among autistic people
- **Professional identity**: Reframing career through autistic strengths
- **Parental identity**: Understanding how autism affects parenting
- **Partner identity**: Renegotiating relationships with new understanding

David, a Black autistic man, found diagnosis complicated his racial identity navigation. Code-switching between Black and white cultural contexts already required enormous energy. Adding autism awareness meant recognizing he'd been triple-masking—hiding autistic traits while performing both professional and cultural expectations. Integration meant finding spaces where all his identities could coexist authentically.

Dealing with Imposter Syndrome

"Am I autistic enough?" This question plagues many newly diagnosed adults, especially those diagnosed later in life after developing extensive coping mechanisms. Imposter syndrome can undermine the validity of your diagnosis and delay accessing needed support.

Common Imposter Syndrome Thoughts:

- "I made eye contact during assessment—maybe I fooled them"
- "Other autistic people seem to struggle more"
- "I have a job/relationship/degree, so I can't really be autistic"
- "Maybe I just wanted to belong somewhere"
- "The psychologist made a mistake"
- "I'm not like media portrayals of autism"

These doubts often intensify when:

- Meeting autistic people with different support needs
- Functioning well in familiar environments
- Comparing yourself to stereotypes
- Others question your diagnosis
- Masking feels successful

Emma's imposter syndrome peaked three months post-diagnosis. She'd joined an autism support group where several members were non-speaking or had obvious support needs. Her ability to maintain employment and live independently made her question her diagnosis validity. The group facilitator, also late-diagnosed, reminded her that autism isn't a competition—her struggles were real regardless of others' experiences.

Combating Imposter Syndrome:

Remember diagnosis criteria: You met clinical criteria for autism. Professionals don't hand out diagnoses carelessly. Your assessment captured your authentic neurology, not momentary performance.

Acknowledge masking costs: Just because you can appear neurotypical doesn't mean it's sustainable or healthy. Consider the energy expenditure, burnout cycles, and mental health impact of constant camouflaging.

Validate your struggles: Compare yourself to neurotypical peers, not other autistic people. Your challenges are real regardless of others' experiences.

Document difficult moments: Imposter syndrome often strikes when you're functioning well. Keep records of struggles to remind yourself why you sought diagnosis.

Connect with similar adults: Find late-diagnosed adults with similar presentations. Shared experiences combat isolation and doubt.

Sharing Your Diagnosis Strategically

Disclosure decisions following adult diagnosis require careful consideration. Unlike children whose parents manage disclosure, you must navigate complex decisions about who to tell, when, and how much to share.

Creating Disclosure Strategies:

Consider these factors for each potential disclosure:

- **Relationship depth**: Closer relationships may warrant more detail
- **Safety assessment**: Will disclosure risk discrimination or harm?
- **Potential benefits**: Could disclosure improve the relationship or situation?
- **Their autism knowledge**: Will education be required?
- **Your energy availability**: Do you have capacity for potential reactions?

Disclosure Circles Model:

Organize disclosure decisions in expanding circles:

Inner Circle - Full Disclosure:

- Intimate partners
- Immediate family (if safe)
- Closest friends
- Your therapist/medical team

Middle Circle - Partial Disclosure:

- Extended family
- Good friends
- Trusted colleagues
- Your manager (for accommodations)

Outer Circle - Strategic Disclosure:

- Acquaintances
- General workplace
- Service providers
- Social communities

No Disclosure - Protected Information:

- Unsafe family members
- Discriminatory environments
- Casual encounters
- Social media (unless chosen)

Crafting Your Disclosure Script:

Different situations require different approaches:

For intimate relationships: "I recently discovered I'm autistic. This explains many of my experiences and needs. I'd like to share what this means for me and our relationship..."

For workplace accommodations: "I have a neurological condition that affects sensory processing and communication. I need some workplace adjustments to perform optimally..."

For casual disclosure: "I'm autistic, which means my brain processes things differently. For me, this looks like..."

Managing Reactions:

People respond to disclosure in various ways:

- **Supportive**: "Thank you for trusting me. How can I help?"
- **Dismissive**: "Everyone's a little autistic" or "You don't look autistic"
- **Curious**: Excessive questions about your experience
- **Skeptical**: Questioning your diagnosis validity
- **Anxious**: Worry about saying the wrong thing

Rebecca's disclosure journey illustrates strategic thinking. She told her partner immediately, needing support processing diagnosis. Her parents required a month of her own processing first, plus printed resources. At work, she disclosed only to HR for accommodations, using "sensory processing differences" rather than autism. Each disclosure was tailored to relationship dynamics and practical needs.

Building Your Support Team

Post-diagnosis life improves dramatically with appropriate support. Building a comprehensive team takes time but provides essential resources for thriving as an autistic adult.

Professional Support Members:

Autism-affirming therapist: Seek therapists who:

- Understand adult autism presentation
- Support neurodiversity perspectives
- Don't try to "fix" autistic traits
- Help with identity integration
- Address autism-related trauma

Psychiatrist (if needed): For co-occurring conditions:

- Anxiety and depression management
- ADHD medication if concurrent
- Sleep disorder treatment
- Trauma-informed approaches

Occupational therapist: Often overlooked for adults:

- Sensory integration strategies
- Executive function supports
- Daily living skills adaptations
- Workplace modifications

Autism coach: Growing field offering:

- Practical life strategies
- Social navigation support
- Career development
- Advocacy skill building

Community Support Networks:

Online communities provide:

- 24/7 peer support access
- Diverse perspectives on autism
- Practical advice from lived experience
- Validation and understanding
- Resource sharing

Local support groups offer:

- In-person connection
- Regular meeting structure
- Facilitated discussions
- Activity-based gatherings
- Advocacy opportunities

Mentorship relationships:

- Other late-diagnosed adults
- Autistic professionals in your field
- Parents of autistic children (if relevant)
- Advocacy leaders

Michael built his support team methodically over two years. Starting with an autism-affirming therapist helped process diagnosis. Adding an occupational therapist addressed sensory needs affecting sleep and work. Joining both online and local autistic communities provided peer support. Finding an autistic mentor in his engineering field transformed his career trajectory. Each addition strengthened his support network.

Family and Friend Allies:

Educating existing relationships creates natural support:

1. **Share resources**: Books, articles, videos about adult autism
2. **Explain your needs**: Specific ways they can support you
3. **Set boundaries**: What comments or behaviors aren't helpful
4. **Appreciate efforts**: Acknowledge their learning journey
5. **Be patient**: Understanding takes time

FAQ: "Do I have to tell everyone?"

No, you absolutely don't have to tell everyone about your autism diagnosis. Disclosure is entirely your choice, and you maintain complete control over who knows, when they learn, and how much detail you share.

Your disclosure rights include:

- Choosing never to disclose to certain people
- Sharing different amounts of information with different people
- Changing your mind about disclosure decisions
- Requesting confidentiality from those you tell
- Disclosing without using the word "autism" if preferred

Factors supporting non-disclosure:

- Workplace discrimination concerns
- Unsafe family dynamics
- Cultural stigma
- Personal privacy preferences
- Energy conservation
- Previous negative experiences

Alternative approaches to full disclosure:

- Describing specific needs without diagnostic labels
- Using terms like "neurodivergent" or "differently wired"
- Focusing on accommodations rather than diagnosis
- Selective trait disclosure as relevant
- Allowing close allies to facilitate understanding

Many adults create nuanced disclosure strategies. Anna tells her immediate family and closest friends about her autism. At work, she requests accommodations for "sensory processing sensitivity" without mentioning autism. With acquaintances, she might mention being "detail-oriented" or "needing routine" without diagnostic disclosure. This graduated approach protects her while meeting practical needs.

Disclosure decisions can change over time. Initial diagnosis often brings pressure to tell everyone immediately. As identity integrates, many adults become more selective and strategic about disclosure. There's no right or wrong approach—only what serves your wellbeing and practical needs.

Key Takeaways

- Post-diagnosis emotions range from relief to grief, all valid parts of processing this life-changing information
- Identity reconstruction involves reframing your entire life story through an autistic lens, integrating this understanding with other aspects of identity
- Imposter syndrome commonly affects late-diagnosed adults but can be countered by remembering diagnosis validity and masking costs
- Disclosure decisions require strategic thinking, considering relationships, safety, and potential benefits
- Building a comprehensive support team of professionals, community members, and educated allies significantly improves post-diagnosis life
- You maintain complete autonomy over disclosure decisions, with no obligation to tell everyone
- Post-diagnosis adjustment takes time—be patient with yourself as you navigate this new understanding

The Journey Continues

Diagnosis marks not an end but a beginning—the start of living authentically as your autistic self. With understanding comes the opportunity to build a life that works with rather than against your neurology. The journey forward involves continued learning, self-advocacy, and community connection as you discover what thriving looks like for you as an autistic adult.

Chapter 7: Workplace Rights and Accommodations

The fluorescent lights hum overhead as you sit at your desk, fighting the familiar sensory overload that makes concentration feel like swimming through molasses. Your coworker's cologne mingles with the break room microwave smell, creating a nauseating combination. The open office chatter builds to an unbearable crescendo. You need accommodations, but asking feels impossible. How do you explain needs that you've spent years hiding? This chapter provides the roadmap for navigating workplace rights, securing accommodations, and building a sustainable career as an autistic adult.

Legal Protections (ADA, Equivalent Laws Globally)

Understanding your legal rights forms the foundation for workplace self-advocacy. While laws vary globally, most developed nations provide some protection for autistic employees. Knowing these protections empowers you to request necessary accommodations without apology.

United States - Americans with Disabilities Act (ADA):

The ADA, enacted in 1990 and amended in 2008, prohibits discrimination against qualified individuals with disabilities in all employment practices (36). For autistic adults, key provisions include:

- **Coverage**: Applies to employers with 15 or more employees
- **Protection scope**: Hiring, firing, advancement, compensation, training
- **Reasonable accommodations**: Required unless causing "undue hardship"

- **Disclosure protection**: Can't be forced to disclose, but must disclose to receive accommodations
- **Retaliation prohibition**: Illegal to punish accommodation requests

Sarah's experience illustrates ADA protection in action. After receiving her autism diagnosis at 35, she requested noise-canceling headphones and written instructions for new tasks at her marketing firm. Her manager initially resisted, calling these "preferences." Sarah provided her diagnosis documentation and ADA information. The company's HR department, recognizing their legal obligations, approved her accommodations within two weeks.

United Kingdom - Equality Act 2010:

The Equality Act provides similar protections to the ADA:

- **Automatic coverage**: Autism qualifies as disability without proving substantial impact
- **Reasonable adjustments**: Employers must remove barriers
- **Anticipatory duty**: Employers should proactively consider needs
- **Protection from harassment**: Covers disability-related bullying
- **Access to Work scheme**: Government funding for accommodations

Canada - Employment Equity Act & Human Rights Act:

Canadian protections include:

- **Duty to accommodate**: Up to "undue hardship"
- **Provincial variations**: Each province has additional protections

- **Broader discrimination definition**: Includes perceived disability
- **Privacy rights**: Strict limits on medical information sharing

European Union - Employment Equality Directive:

EU-wide protections with country-specific implementation:

- **Reasonable accommodation requirement**: Across all member states
- **Positive action allowed**: Employers can favor disabled candidates
- **Varying enforcement**: Country-dependent effectiveness
- **Cross-border protections**: Rights travel within EU

Australia - Disability Discrimination Act 1992:

Australian law provides:

- **Inherent requirements test**: Must be able to perform essential job functions
- **Reasonable adjustment obligation**: Similar to other nations
- **Positive duty**: Employers must eliminate discrimination
- **Conciliation focus**: Emphasis on resolution over litigation

Understanding your local laws matters because enforcement, definitions, and processes vary significantly. Research your specific jurisdiction's protections, enforcement agencies, and complaint procedures.

Reasonable Accommodation Examples

Accommodations aren't special privileges—they're modifications that enable equal access to employment.

Understanding the range of possible accommodations helps you identify what might support your success.

Communication Accommodations:

- Written instructions instead of verbal
- Email communication preferred over phone calls
- Agenda provided before meetings
- Permission to use AAC devices if needed
- Regular written feedback instead of impromptu reviews
- Clear, direct communication expectations

Michael, a software developer, struggled with verbal processing during fast-paced meetings. His accommodations included receiving meeting agendas 24 hours in advance, permission to process questions before responding, and follow-up emails summarizing verbal discussions. These simple modifications transformed his meeting participation from stressful performances to productive contributions.

Sensory Accommodations:

- Noise-canceling headphones or earplugs
- Modified lighting (lamps instead of fluorescents)
- Fragrance-free workplace policies
- Private workspace or cubicle walls
- Permission to take sensory breaks
- Flexible dress code for sensory needs

Schedule and Structure Accommodations:

- Consistent work schedule
- Advance notice of changes
- Written daily/weekly schedules
- Flexible hours to avoid rush hour
- Work-from-home options
- Regular breaks for regulation

Task and Workload Accommodations:

- Breaking large projects into smaller steps
- Written prioritization of assignments
- Consistent task assignment methods
- Extended deadlines when possible
- Reduced interruptions during focus work
- Modified training approaches

Jennifer's accommodation journey shows creative solutions. As a graphic designer, she excelled at visual work but struggled with client interactions. Her accommodations included a client communication template, permission to have a colleague present during client calls for support, and shifting her role to focus more on design production than client management. Her productivity soared when her role aligned with her strengths.

Environmental Accommodations:

- Assigned parking spot (same location daily)
- Consistent workspace (no hot-desking)
- Temperature control access
- Ability to personalize workspace
- Access to quiet spaces
- Natural light exposure options

Social and Meeting Accommodations:

- Exemption from non-essential social events
- Alternative team-building participation
- Video off option for virtual meetings
- Structured meeting roles
- Social scripts for common interactions
- Buddy system for workplace navigation

Disclosure Decisions and Scripts

Deciding if, when, and how to disclose your autism at work ranks among the most challenging aspects of workplace navigation. No universal answer exists—each situation requires careful consideration of multiple factors.

Disclosure Decision Framework:

Consider these elements when making disclosure decisions:

1. **Legal need**: Accommodations require some disclosure
2. **Workplace culture**: How disability-friendly is your environment?
3. **Job security**: Your position stability affects risk tolerance
4. **Support needs**: Can you function without accommodations?
5. **Career goals**: Will disclosure impact advancement?
6. **Personal comfort**: Your readiness for potential reactions

Levels of Disclosure:

Minimal Disclosure: "I have a neurological condition that affects..."

- Provides legal protection
- Maintains privacy
- Focuses on needs, not labels
- Reduces stigma risk

Partial Disclosure: "I'm neurodivergent and need..."

- Indicates brain differences
- Avoids specific diagnosis
- Creates community connection
- Allows education opportunities

Full Disclosure: "I'm autistic, which means..."

- Complete transparency
- Enables full advocacy
- Risks maximum stigma
- Allows authentic presentation

Disclosure Scripts for Different Scenarios:

To HR for Accommodations: "I have a disability covered under the ADA and need to discuss reasonable accommodations. I have documentation from my healthcare provider. My condition affects sensory processing and communication. I've identified specific accommodations that would help me perform my job optimally."

To Direct Supervisor: "I wanted to share that I've recently been diagnosed with autism spectrum disorder. This doesn't change my ability to do my job, but it does mean I work best with certain supports in place. I've already spoken with HR about formal accommodations, but I wanted you to understand why I might need things like written instructions or quiet workspace."

To Colleagues (if choosing to share): "I'm autistic, which means my brain processes information differently. You might notice I wear headphones to manage sound sensitivity or take notes during verbal instructions. These strategies help me do my best work. I'm happy to answer questions if you're curious about autism."

David's disclosure strategy evolved over time. Initially, he disclosed only to HR, requesting accommodations for "sensory processing disorder." After positive experiences with his immediate team, he shared his autism diagnosis with his supervisor, who became a strong advocate. Eventually, he felt comfortable being openly autistic at work, even presenting about neurodiversity during diversity week.

Self-Advocacy Strategies

Effective self-advocacy transforms workplace experience from daily struggle to sustainable success. Building these skills takes practice but yields long-term benefits for your career and wellbeing.

Know Your Value: Document your contributions:

- Projects completed successfully
- Skills you bring to the team
- Problems you've solved
- Efficiency improvements you've made
- Unique perspectives you offer

This documentation serves dual purposes: building confidence and providing evidence during accommodation discussions.

Build Your Business Case: Frame accommodations as business benefits:

- "Noise-canceling headphones will increase my productivity by 40%"
- "Written instructions reduce error rates and revision time"
- "Flexible hours mean I work during my peak performance times"
- "Remote work eliminates commute sensory stress, improving focus"

Create Allies: Strategic relationship building:

- Identify neurodiversity-friendly colleagues
- Connect with other disabled employees
- Build relationships before needing support
- Offer reciprocal support to allies
- Join or create employee resource groups

Document Everything: Maintain thorough records:

- Accommodation requests and responses
- Performance reviews and feedback
- Discriminatory incidents if they occur
- Medical documentation
- Email communications about needs

Lisa learned documentation's importance the hard way. Her initial verbal accommodation requests were "forgotten" by management. She began email follow-ups after every conversation, creating paper trails. When a new manager tried to revoke her accommodations, her documentation protected her rights.

Practice Boundaries: Setting workplace boundaries:

- "I need to finish this task before switching to another"
- "I'm not available for impromptu meetings—please schedule"
- "I take lunch alone to recharge for afternoon productivity"
- "I communicate better through email than phone calls"

Know When to Escalate: Escalation pathway:

1. Direct conversation with immediate supervisor
2. Formal request to HR with documentation
3. Internal complaint process if needed
4. External agency complaint (EEOC, equivalent)
5. Legal consultation for serious violations

Career Considerations

Autism impacts career development in unique ways. Understanding these influences helps you make strategic decisions aligned with both your needs and ambitions.

Choosing Autism-Compatible Careers:

While autistic people succeed in every field, certain careers align well with common autistic strengths:

Detail-Oriented Fields:

- Quality assurance testing
- Research and analysis
- Accounting and bookkeeping
- Technical writing
- Laboratory work
- Archival and library science

Pattern Recognition Roles:

- Data analysis
- Cybersecurity
- Scientific research
- Music composition
- Programming
- Epidemiology

Systematic Thinking Positions:

- Engineering disciplines
- Mathematics
- Logic-based fields
- Process improvement
- Systems administration
- Urban planning

Special Interest Alignment: The key is matching careers to your specific interests and strengths rather than generic "autism-friendly" lists.

Tom spent years in retail management, burning out repeatedly from constant social demands and sensory chaos. After diagnosis at 38, he transitioned to database administration—a role utilizing his pattern recognition skills while minimizing problematic sensory and social elements. His career satisfaction transformed completely.

Managing Career Transitions:

Career changes post-diagnosis require strategic planning:

1. Assess current role sustainability
2. Identify transferable skills
3. Research accommodation availability in new fields
4. Build skills gradually while employed
5. Network within neurodiversity-friendly companies
6. Consider disclosure timing carefully

Advancement Strategies:

Climbing career ladders while autistic:

- Seek mentors who understand neurodiversity
- Build expertise in specialized areas
- Document achievements meticulously
- Request advancement criteria in writing
- Negotiate role modifications with promotions
- Consider lateral moves for better fit

Entrepreneurship Option:

Some autistic adults find self-employment ideal:

- Complete environmental control
- Work aligned with special interests
- Flexible scheduling
- No disclosure decisions
- Direct correlation between effort and reward
- Ability to build business around strengths

FAQ: "Should I tell my employer?"

This question has no universal answer. Your decision depends on multiple personal factors, and what's right for someone else might not suit your situation.

Reasons to disclose:

- You need accommodations to perform effectively
- Your workplace culture embraces neurodiversity
- Masking exhausts you unsustainably
- You want to advocate for autism acceptance
- Legal protections require disclosure
- Authenticity improves your wellbeing

Reasons not to disclose:

- You function well without accommodations
- Your workplace shows discrimination signs
- Job security concerns exist
- Stigma might limit opportunities
- You prefer privacy about medical information
- Previous negative experiences inform caution

Middle ground approaches: Many adults find creative middle grounds:

- Disclosing needs without diagnostic labels
- Sharing with trusted colleagues but not broadly
- Disclosing to HR but not supervisors
- Using general terms like "neurodivergent"
- Disclosing after establishing strong performance
- Partial disclosure focusing on specific traits

Remember: disclosure isn't permanent or all-or-nothing. You can:

- Start with minimal disclosure and expand later
- Disclose to different people at different levels
- Change your approach as circumstances shift
- Retract disclosure isn't possible, but you can control ongoing information
- Learn from each disclosure experience

Maria's journey illustrates disclosure evolution. She spent two years at her company masking intensely before diagnosis. Post-diagnosis, she disclosed only to HR for accommodations. After six months of successful accommodations, she told her supportive supervisor. Eventually, she became comfortable being openly autistic, even leading the company's neurodiversity initiatives. Her gradual approach allowed comfort building at each stage.

Key Takeaways

- Legal protections exist globally for autistic employees, though specific rights and processes vary by location
- Reasonable accommodations range from communication modifications to environmental changes, all designed to enable equal employment access
- Disclosure decisions require careful consideration of workplace culture, personal needs, and career goals
- Self-advocacy skills build through practice and include knowing your value, building allies, and maintaining documentation
- Career planning benefits from understanding autism's impact on job fit and advancement strategies
- Disclosure decisions aren't permanent or universal—you control your narrative and can adjust approaches over time
- Success comes from aligning work environments with autistic needs rather than forcing unsustainable adaptations

Preparing for Academic Success

The workplace represents just one arena where autistic adults navigate disclosure and accommodation decisions. Educational settings present their own unique challenges and opportunities. The next chapter examines how to secure academic accommodations, develop effective study strategies, and manage the sensory and social demands of higher education as an autistic learner.

Chapter 8: Educational Accommodations

Returning to education as an adult—or continuing education post-diagnosis—means navigating academic systems with new self-awareness. The lecture hall's fluorescent glare, the chaos of group projects, the executive function demands of managing multiple courses simultaneously—these challenges that once seemed like personal failures now make sense through an autistic lens. This chapter guides you through securing educational accommodations, developing autism-aligned study strategies, and creating sustainable academic success.

Rights in Higher Education

Educational rights for autistic students extend beyond childhood, though many adults don't realize these protections continue through higher education. Understanding your rights empowers you to access support without shame or apology.

United States - Section 504 and ADA:

Two federal laws protect autistic students in higher education:

Section 504 of the Rehabilitation Act (1973) prohibits discrimination in any program receiving federal funding—including most colleges and universities (37).

The Americans with Disabilities Act (ADA) extends protections to private institutions not covered by Section 504 (38).

Key differences from K-12 education:

- **No IEP/504 Plan transfers**: Must establish new accommodations

- **Self-advocacy required**: Institution won't identify your needs
- **Documentation necessary**: Must prove disability impact
- **"Reasonable" standard**: Accommodations can't fundamentally alter programs
- **Equal access, not success**: Right to access, not guaranteed outcomes

Rachel discovered these differences dramatically. Throughout K-12, her school initiated support services. Arriving at university, she expected similar proactive support. Instead, she struggled for an entire semester before learning she needed to self-identify to Disability Services and provide documentation.

International Educational Rights:

United Kingdom:

- Equality Act 2010 covers higher education
- Disabled Students' Allowance provides funding
- Anticipatory reasonable adjustments required
- No means testing for support

Canada:

- Provincial human rights legislation applies
- Duty to accommodate to "undue hardship"
- Bursaries available for students with disabilities
- Varies significantly by province

Australia:

- Disability Discrimination Act covers education
- Disability Standards for Education 2005
- Inherent requirement concept applies
- Support funding through various programs

European Union:

- UN Convention on Rights of Persons with Disabilities
- Country-specific implementation varies
- Erasmus+ includes disability support
- Cross-border study accommodations

Understanding your specific country's framework matters because processes, funding, and available accommodations differ significantly.

Accommodation Request Process

Securing academic accommodations requires systematic approach and persistence. Unlike workplace accommodations, educational accommodations often involve multiple offices and stricter documentation requirements.

Step 1: Locate Disability Services

Every institution names their office differently:

- Disability Services
- Accessibility Resources
- Student Support Services
- Academic Accommodations Office
- Equity and Inclusion Center

Contact them before enrollment when possible. Early connection allows planning time.

Step 2: Gather Documentation

Most institutions require:

- **Diagnostic documentation**: Recent evaluation (usually within 3-5 years)

- **Functional impact statement**: How autism affects academic performance
- **Accommodation history**: Previous accommodations received
- **Provider recommendations**: Specific accommodation suggestions

James faced documentation challenges when returning to school at 40. His childhood diagnosis documentation was deemed "too old." He needed new evaluation costing $2,000 before accessing accommodations. Planning for this expense and time requirement proves essential.

Step 3: Initial Meeting

Prepare for your intake appointment:

- List all functional limitations
- Bring documentation organized chronologically
- Prepare to explain autism's academic impact
- Know what accommodations you want
- Ask about appeals processes
- Request written accommodation plans

Step 4: Negotiate Accommodations

Common academic accommodations include:

Testing Accommodations:

- Extended time (typically 1.5x or 2x)
- Reduced distraction environment
- Breaks during exams
- Alternative test formats
- Clarification of questions
- Use of technology

Classroom Accommodations:

- Recording lectures
- Note-taking assistance
- Preferential seating
- Attendance flexibility
- Fidget/stim tools allowed
- Advance access to materials

Assignment Accommodations:

- Extended deadlines
- Alternative assignment formats
- Broken-down project steps
- Written instructions for all assignments
- Exemption from group work
- Regular check-ins with instructors

Communication Accommodations:

- Email contact preferred
- Written feedback
- Clear rubrics
- Advance notice of changes
- Direct communication style accepted
- AAC device use if needed

Environmental Accommodations:

- Access to quiet study spaces
- Housing accommodations
- Lighting modifications
- Fragrance-free spaces
- Consistent classroom locations
- Sensory break permissions

Maria's accommodation negotiation illustrates the process. She initially received only extended test time. Through self-advocacy, she added: permission to type instead of handwrite, access to a private testing room, and exemption from surprise "pop quizzes" that triggered panic. Each semester, she refined her accommodations based on experience.

Step 5: Implementation

After approval:

1. Obtain official accommodation letters
2. Meet with each instructor individually
3. Discuss specific implementation
4. Clarify any confusion about accommodations
5. Establish communication preferences
6. Document all conversations

Step 6: Monitor and Adjust

Accommodations aren't static:

- Evaluate effectiveness each term
- Request modifications as needed
- Document what works and what doesn't
- Build relationships with disability services
- Know your appeal rights
- Advocate for improvements

Study Strategies for Autistic Learners

Traditional study advice often fails autistic students. Developing strategies aligned with autistic learning styles transforms academic experience from struggle to success.

Working with Autistic Strengths:

Pattern Recognition:

- Create visual maps showing concept relationships
- Use color-coding systems for information categories
- Build personal databases of course information
- Look for systematic rules underlying material
- Connect new information to existing frameworks

Detail Focus:

- Master foundational concepts thoroughly before advancing
- Create comprehensive notes capturing all details
- Use specific examples to understand general principles
- Build understanding from bottom-up
- Maintain running lists of questions

Special Interests Integration:

- Connect course material to interests when possible
- Choose research topics within interest areas
- Use interest-based metaphors for difficult concepts
- Create projects combining courses with interests
- Find interest-aligned study partners

David studied computer science but struggled with required humanities courses. He began relating every humanities concept to programming concepts—viewing history as debugging human systems, analyzing literature like code structure. This translation through special interest improved his grades dramatically.

Managing Executive Function:

Time Management Systems:

- Use digital calendars with multiple alerts
- Break assignments into tiny, specific steps

- Set artificial early deadlines
- Use time-tracking apps to build awareness
- Create routine study schedules
- Plan backwards from due dates

Organization Structures:

- One consistent system across all courses
- Digital tools for easy searching
- Color-coded folders/notebooks
- Templates for common assignments
- Checklists for multi-step processes
- Regular system maintenance time

Task Initiation Strategies:

- Environmental cues for study time
- Body doubling (studying alongside others)
- Pomodoro technique with rewards
- Starting with easiest/most interesting part
- External accountability partners
- Removing all barriers to starting

Sensory Considerations for Studying:

Create optimal study environments:

- **Lighting**: Natural light or warm lamps
- **Sound**: White noise, nature sounds, or silence
- **Temperature**: Consistent and comfortable
- **Seating**: Supportive with movement options
- **Stimming**: Fidget tools readily available
- **Breaks**: Regular sensory regulation time

Lisa discovered her ideal study environment through experimentation. She studies best at 5 AM in her apartment's breakfast nook, wearing noise-canceling headphones playing brown noise, with her weighted lap pad, surrounded by her color-coded materials. This precise environment enables four-hour focus sessions.

Managing Academic Stress

Academic environments create unique stressors for autistic students. Understanding and managing these pressures prevents burnout and enables sustained success.

Common Academic Stressors:

Social Demands:

- Group project navigation
- Class participation requirements
- Networking expectations
- Study group dynamics
- Presentation requirements
- Office hours interactions

Sensory Challenges:

- Crowded lecture halls
- Fluorescent classroom lighting
- Food court chaos
- Library study areas
- Campus transportation
- Dormitory living

Executive Function Overload:

- Multiple course management
- Competing deadlines
- Schedule changes
- Registration processes
- Administrative requirements

- Life balance demands

Communication Difficulties:

- Understanding assignment expectations
- Interpreting feedback
- Asking for help
- Email management
- Peer interactions
- Professor relationships

Stress Management Strategies:

Preventive Measures:

1. Build buffer time into all schedules
2. Create consistent routines
3. Maintain regular sleep schedules
4. Plan sensory regulation activities
5. Limit course loads if possible
6. Choose professors carefully using reviews

Active Coping Techniques:

- Daily stimming sessions
- Regular special interest time
- Movement breaks between classes
- Mindfulness adapted for autism
- Journaling or creative expression
- Connection with autistic peers

Crisis Management Plans: When overwhelm hits:

1. Pre-written emails requesting extensions
2. Identified safe spaces on campus
3. Emergency contact list
4. Shutdown recovery protocols

5. Missing class contingency plans
6. Support network activation steps

Tom's stress management evolved through trial and error. Initially, he pushed through mounting stress until complete shutdown. Now, he monitors early warning signs—increased stimming, food texture sensitivity, word-finding difficulties. When these appear, he implements his "pressure release protocol": canceling non-essential commitments, spending entire weekend in special interest activities, and preemptively communicating with professors about potential needs.

Online Learning Considerations

Online education offers unique advantages and challenges for autistic learners. The pandemic-driven shift to digital learning revealed both accessibility improvements and new barriers.

Online Learning Advantages:

Environmental Control:

- Study in sensory-friendly spaces
- Eliminate commute stress
- Control lighting and sound
- Wear comfortable clothing
- Stim freely during lectures
- Take breaks as needed

Communication Benefits:

- Written discussion forums
- Time to process before responding
- Reduced real-time social demands
- Clear digital assignment submissions
- Recorded lectures for review
- Asynchronous participation options

Executive Function Supports:

- Digital organization systems
- Automated reminders
- Clear assignment tracking
- Consistent interface
- Searchable content
- Flexible scheduling

Online Learning Challenges:

Technology Barriers:

- Platform navigation difficulties
- Multiple software requirements
- Technical troubleshooting stress
- Internet reliability needs
- Camera/microphone anxiety
- Digital eye strain

Communication Issues:

- Lack of routine structure
- Difficulty reading digital social cues
- Zoom fatigue from video calls
- Delayed instructor responses
- Peer connection challenges
- Reduced accommodation visibility

Strategies for Online Success:

1. **Create rigid structure**: Without campus routines, build your own
2. **Optimize technology**: Invest in quality equipment reducing frustration
3. **Communicate proactively**: Over-communicate with instructors

4. **Build peer connections**: Find alternative ways to connect
5. **Maintain boundaries**: Separate study space from living space
6. **Use accessibility features**: Captions, transcripts, playback speed

Sarah thrived in online learning after initial adjustment. She created a dedicated study corner with perfect lighting, established strict daily routines, and used the chat function for class participation instead of speaking. Her grades improved compared to in-person classes, though she missed library study spaces.

FAQ: "Can I get accommodations without formal diagnosis?"

This depends entirely on your institution and location. Some schools accept alternative documentation, while others require specific diagnostic proof.

Alternatives to formal diagnosis:

- **Psychoeducational evaluations**: May identify learning differences
- **Mental health provider letters**: Describing functional limitations
- **Medical documentation**: Of related conditions (anxiety, sensory issues)
- **Previous accommodation history**: From other institutions
- **Functional assessment**: Focusing on needs rather than diagnosis

Institutions more likely to be flexible:

- Community colleges

- Online universities
- Continuing education programs
- Certificate programs
- International institutions
- Progressive universities

Strategies without formal documentation:

1. Meet with disability services anyway—policies may be flexible
2. Work directly with understanding professors
3. Use informal accommodations (sitting near doors, recording lectures)
4. Build support networks with peers
5. Access tutoring and academic support services
6. Utilize technology solutions independently

The documentation dilemma: Many autistic adults face catch-22 situations: needing accommodations to succeed academically but unable to afford diagnostic assessment. Some strategies:

- Research sliding-scale assessment options
- Check if student health provides evaluations
- Apply for diagnostic scholarships
- Consider payment plans for assessment
- Explore whether partial documentation suffices
- Document functional needs thoroughly

Michael navigated this challenge creatively. Unable to afford full autism assessment, he obtained documentation from his therapist describing sensory processing difficulties and executive function challenges. Combined with his previous ADHD diagnosis, this provided enough documentation for basic accommodations while he saved for comprehensive evaluation.

The self-advocacy required may feel daunting, but many autistic students successfully obtain accommodations through persistence and creative documentation. Start conversations with disability services—they may surprise you with flexibility.

Key Takeaways

- Educational rights continue through higher education, though processes differ significantly from K-12 special education
- Securing accommodations requires self-advocacy, documentation, and systematic navigation of institutional processes
- Academic accommodations range from testing modifications to environmental adjustments, tailored to individual needs
- Study strategies aligned with autistic learning styles leverage strengths while supporting challenges
- Managing academic stress requires preventive measures, active coping techniques, and crisis planning
- Online learning presents both advantages and challenges requiring specific strategies for success
- Accommodations without formal diagnosis may be possible through alternative documentation and creative advocacy

Healthcare Navigation Ahead

Academic success provides one foundation for adult life, but maintaining physical and mental health requires equally careful navigation. The next chapter examines how to find autism-informed healthcare providers, adapt therapeutic approaches for autistic needs, and manage the complex intersection of autism with co-occurring conditions.

Chapter 9: Healthcare and Therapy Options

The waiting room's flickering fluorescent light triggers familiar pre-meltdown warning signs. The receptionist's perfume mingles with cleaning chemicals, creating an overwhelming sensory assault. You're here seeking help, but the healthcare environment itself becomes a barrier. For autistic adults, finding appropriate healthcare means more than locating providers—it requires finding professionals who understand how autism affects every aspect of health and healing. This chapter guides you through building a healthcare team that works with, not against, your neurology.

Finding Autism-Informed Providers

The search for healthcare providers who understand adult autism often feels like hunting for unicorns. Many professionals received no training about autism beyond outdated stereotypes, if any training at all. Building an effective healthcare team requires strategic searching and careful vetting.

Identifying Knowledgeable Providers:

Start your search with these strategies:

Professional Directories:

- Autism organization provider lists
- Neurodiversity-affirming therapist directories
- LGBTQ+ friendly providers (often more neurodiversity aware)
- Integrative medicine practitioners
- Providers listing autism as a specialty

Community Recommendations:

- Local autistic adult groups
- Online community recommendations
- Parent groups (for family practice references)
- Disability service organizations
- University-affiliated clinics

Vetting Questions to Ask:

Before scheduling, interview potential providers:

1. "What experience do you have with autistic adults?"
2. "How do you view autism—as a disorder to treat or a neurological difference?"
3. "Are you familiar with autistic masking and burnout?"
4. "How do you accommodate sensory needs in your practice?"
5. "What's your understanding of autism beyond stereotypes?"
6. "Will you write letters supporting accommodations?"

Dr. Chen's search illustrates the process. After three dismissive physicians told her she "didn't look autistic," she developed a screening system. She called offices asking specific questions about autism understanding. The fourth practice she contacted had a nurse practitioner whose son was autistic. This provider understood sensory accommodations, communication differences, and the importance of routine—transforming Dr. Chen's healthcare experience.

Red Flags to Avoid:

Certain responses indicate providers to skip:

- "I treat many children with autism" (without adult experience)
- "You seem too high-functioning to need accommodations"

- "Have you tried just being less rigid?"
- "Autism is overdiagnosed these days"
- Recommending cure-focused treatments
- Dismissing sensory experiences
- Using functioning labels

Building Your Healthcare Team:

A complete team might include:

Primary Care Provider (PCP):

- Manages overall health
- Provides accommodation letters
- Monitors medication interactions
- Addresses autism-related health issues
- Coordinates specialist referrals

Mental Health Professionals:

- Psychiatrist for medication management
- Therapist for ongoing support
- Neuropsychologist for cognitive assessment
- Trauma specialist if needed

Specialists as Needed:

- Neurologist for seizures/migraines
- Gastroenterologist for GI issues
- Sleep specialist for sleep disorders
- Dietitian familiar with ARFID
- Occupational therapist for daily living skills

Creating Provider Communication Strategies:

Once you find good providers, optimize communication:

1. **Request appointment modifications**:
   - First or last appointment slots
   - Extended appointment times
   - Dimmed lighting options
   - Email communication between visits
   - Written visit summaries
2. **Prepare for appointments**:
   - Write questions in advance
   - Bring sensory tools
   - Use communication apps if needed
   - Request specific exam modifications
   - Bring support person if helpful
3. **Educate your providers**:
   - Share articles about adult autism
   - Explain your specific needs
   - Provide written accommodation requests
   - Give feedback about what helps
   - Build collaborative relationships

Therapy Approaches (CBT Adaptations, DBT)

Traditional therapy approaches often require modification for autistic adults. Understanding how different therapeutic modalities can be adapted helps you find effective mental health support.

Cognitive Behavioral Therapy (CBT) Adaptations:

Standard CBT assumes neurotypical processing and can inadvertently invalidate autistic experiences. Effective adaptations include (39):

Concrete Language:

- Avoid metaphors and abstract concepts
- Use visual aids and written materials
- Provide specific examples

- Break down complex ideas
- Define all terminology clearly

Sensory Considerations:

- Address sensory triggers affecting mood
- Include sensory regulation in coping plans
- Recognize sensory overload vs. anxiety
- Incorporate stimming as regulation tool
- Modify therapy environment

Executive Function Supports:

- Provide session structure predictably
- Write down homework assignments
- Break tasks into tiny steps
- Use checklists and reminders
- Build on existing routines

Autism-Specific Modifications:

- Challenge "correct" social behavior assumptions
- Validate different communication styles
- Address masking and burnout
- Include special interests in therapy
- Recognize autism-related trauma

Sarah's therapy journey demonstrates adaptation needs. Her first therapist used standard CBT, challenging her "irrational" thoughts about social situations. But her social anxiety stemmed from genuine communication differences, not distorted thinking. Her second therapist adapted CBT to address real social navigation challenges while validating her different social needs. This shift from "fixing" to supporting transformed therapy effectiveness.

Dialectical Behavior Therapy (DBT) for Autistic Adults:

DBT's structured approach and skills focus often suits autistic learning styles (40):

Distress Tolerance Skills:

- TIPP adapted for sensory needs
- Stimming as self-soothing
- Special interests for distraction
- Sensory kits for crisis management
- Routine as comfort tool

Emotion Regulation:

- Identifying emotions through body sensations
- Understanding alexithymia impacts
- Tracking patterns systematically
- Using visual emotion scales
- Building sensory regulation plans

Interpersonal Effectiveness:

- Scripts for common situations
- Direct communication validation
- Boundary setting strategies
- Social energy management
- Relationship maintenance systems

Mindfulness Adaptations:

- Movement-based mindfulness
- Special interest meditation
- Sensory-focused practices
- Structured observation exercises
- Pattern-recognition mindfulness

Other Therapeutic Approaches:

Acceptance and Commitment Therapy (ACT):

- Values-based framework suits autistic thinking
- Accepts rather than changes differences
- Psychological flexibility helpful for rigidity
- Mindfulness components adaptable

EMDR for Trauma:

- Bilateral stimulation through preferred sensory channel
- Adapted for autistic processing speed
- Addresses autism-related trauma
- Modifications for eye contact discomfort

Somatic Therapies:

- Body-based approaches for alexithymia
- Sensorimotor psychotherapy
- Polyvagal theory applications
- Movement therapies

Michael found success with adapted DBT after years of ineffective talk therapy. The structured skills training appealed to his systematic thinking. His therapist modified interpersonal effectiveness modules to include autism-specific scenarios like disclosing diagnosis at work and managing small talk. The combination of validation and practical skills finally provided useful support.

Occupational Therapy for Adults

Occupational therapy (OT) remains underutilized for autistic adults despite offering practical support for daily living challenges. Adult OT focuses on functional skills and environmental modifications rather than childhood development goals.

Areas OT Can Address:

Sensory Integration and Regulation:

- Comprehensive sensory assessment
- Personalized sensory diet development
- Environmental modification recommendations
- Sensory tool selection and use
- Regulation strategy development

Executive Function Support:

- Task analysis and modification
- Organization system development
- Time management strategies
- Planning and prioritization tools
- Routine development and maintenance

Activities of Daily Living (ADLs):

- Meal planning and preparation
- Hygiene routine optimization
- Household management systems
- Financial management strategies
- Healthcare navigation skills

Fine and Gross Motor Skills:

- Handwriting alternatives
- Adaptive equipment recommendations
- Coordination exercises
- Workplace ergonomics
- Movement planning strategies

Social and Communication Skills:

- Workplace interaction strategies

- Community navigation planning
- Advocacy skill development
- Relationship maintenance systems
- Communication tool selection

Jennifer's OT experience transformed her daily life. At 34, she struggled with meal preparation, household organization, and sensory overload. Her occupational therapist conducted comprehensive assessment, identifying specific barriers. Together, they developed systems: meal planning templates accounting for texture preferences, cleaning routines broken into manageable chunks, and a personalized sensory kit for community outings. Six months later, Jennifer lived independently for the first time.

Finding Adult OT Services:

Locating OTs experienced with autistic adults requires persistence:

- Contact outpatient rehabilitation centers
- Search for sensory integration certified OTs
- Check university OT programs for clinics
- Ask autism organizations for referrals
- Consider telehealth OT services
- Look for private practice specialists

Making OT Accessible:

Insurance coverage varies, but strategies exist:

- Get physician referral emphasizing functional limitations
- Document specific ADL challenges
- Request evaluation to establish medical necessity
- Appeal coverage denials with research
- Consider intensive short-term intervention
- Explore sliding scale options

Managing Co-occurring Conditions

Autistic adults experience higher rates of various health conditions. Understanding these connections helps you advocate for appropriate treatment that considers autism's impact (41).

Common Co-occurring Mental Health Conditions:

Anxiety Disorders:

- Often stems from sensory overload and social demands
- May manifest differently (shutdown vs. panic)
- Requires autism-informed treatment
- Sensory triggers need addressing
- Social anxiety vs. communication differences

Depression:

- Can result from chronic masking
- Autistic burnout misdiagnosed as depression
- Loss of special interests key symptom
- Requires careful medication monitoring
- Environmental factors crucial

ADHD:

- High co-occurrence rate (50-70%)
- Overlapping executive function challenges
- Combined presentation affects treatment
- Medication responses may differ
- Need integrated support approach

Trauma and PTSD:

- Higher trauma exposure rates
- Autism-related trauma common
- Different trauma responses

- Sensory aspects of trauma
- Need specialized treatment approaches

David's diagnostic journey illustrates complexity. Initially diagnosed with anxiety and depression, treatment barely helped. Years later, autism diagnosis revealed his anxiety stemmed from sensory overload and social exhaustion. Adding ADHD diagnosis explained executive function struggles. Finally, addressing autism-related trauma from decades of forced compliance completed the picture. Integrated treatment addressing all conditions finally brought relief.

Common Physical Health Conditions:

Gastrointestinal Issues:

- IBS and inflammatory conditions common
- Sensory eating restrictions impact nutrition
- Stress affects gut health
- Need gastroenterologist familiar with autism
- Dietary modifications considering sensory needs

Sleep Disorders:

- Circadian rhythm differences
- Sensory barriers to sleep
- Anxiety affecting sleep
- Melatonin production differences
- Need comprehensive sleep assessment

Connective Tissue Disorders:

- Ehlers-Danlos syndrome correlation
- Joint hypermobility common
- Proprioceptive differences
- Chronic pain management needs
- Physical therapy adaptations required

Seizure Disorders:

- Higher epilepsy rates
- Sensory seizures possible
- Medication sensitivity common
- Need specialized monitoring
- Lifestyle modifications important

Integrated Treatment Approaches:

Effective treatment considers all conditions:

1. **Find providers who understand interactions**
2. **Coordinate between specialists**
3. **Monitor medication interactions carefully**
4. **Address root causes, not just symptoms**
5. **Consider alternative treatments**
6. **Modify treatments for autism**

Medication Considerations

Medication management for autistic adults requires careful consideration of sensory sensitivities, processing differences, and atypical responses. Many autistic people experience different medication effects than neurotypical populations.

Sensory Considerations:

Medication Format:

- Texture aversions affecting pills
- Liquid medication taste issues
- Patch adhesive sensitivities
- Injection anxiety
- Alternative delivery methods

Starting Medications:

Autistic adults often benefit from:

- Starting below standard doses
- Slower titration schedules
- Single medication changes
- Detailed side effect tracking
- Clear discontinuation plans

Lisa's medication journey required patience. Standard SSRI doses caused intense side effects. Her psychiatrist started at pediatric doses, increasing slowly over months. This approach revealed her therapeutic dose was one-third typical adult dosing. The slow titration prevented intolerable side effects while achieving benefit.

Common Medication Sensitivities:

Heightened Side Effects:

- Gastrointestinal distress
- Sleep disturbances
- Sensory amplification
- Emotional blunting
- Cognitive fog

Paradoxical Reactions:

- Stimulants causing calm
- Sedatives causing agitation
- Unexpected mood changes
- Opposite intended effects

Medication Classes and Considerations:

Antidepressants:

- SSRIs may help anxiety but worsen sensory issues

- SNRIs might affect executive function
- Careful monitoring for activation
- Sexual side effects impact relationships

Anti-anxiety Medications:

- Benzodiazepines risk dependence
- Beta-blockers for physical symptoms
- Buspirone as alternative
- Consider situational use

ADHD Medications:

- May improve executive function
- Monitor for increased anxiety
- Appetite/sleep effects significant
- Both stimulant/non-stimulant options

Mood Stabilizers:

- For emotional dysregulation
- Monitor cognitive effects
- Blood level monitoring challenging
- Sensory side effects possible

Sleep Medications:

- Melatonin often first choice
- Prescription options if needed
- Address underlying causes
- Avoid long-term dependence

Communication with Prescribers:

Optimize medication management:

1. **Keep detailed symptom logs**

2. **Report all side effects**
3. **Ask about autism-specific research**
4. **Request genetic testing if available**
5. **Discuss non-medication alternatives**
6. **Never stop medications abruptly**

Chapter FAQ: "Do I need therapy if I'm doing fine?"

"Doing fine" means different things to different people. Many autistic adults maintain function through unsustainable coping mechanisms. Consider therapy if:

Hidden Struggles Exist:

- Constant exhaustion from masking
- Regular burnout cycles
- Relationship difficulties
- Employment instability
- Daily living challenges
- Chronic stress or anxiety

Preventive Support Helps:

- Building sustainable strategies
- Processing diagnosis
- Developing self-advocacy skills
- Creating support networks
- Planning for transitions
- Understanding your neurology

Specific Goals:

- Reducing masking safely
- Managing life transitions
- Healing from trauma
- Improving relationships
- Building executive function

- Developing coping strategies

Tom thought he was "fine" - good job, stable relationship, independent living. But beneath the surface, he white-knuckled through each day, collapsed every weekend, and experienced quarterly burnouts. Therapy helped him recognize unsustainable patterns and build genuinely sustainable approaches. "Fine" transformed from survival to thriving.

Therapy isn't just for crisis:

Consider therapy as:

- Neurology education
- Skill building
- Identity exploration
- Preventive maintenance
- Growth opportunity
- Self-understanding tool

Alternatives to Traditional Therapy:

- Autism coaching
- Peer support groups
- Online communities
- Self-help resources
- Workshops and classes
- Mentorship relationships

The decision remains personal. Some autistic adults thrive without professional support, using community resources and self-knowledge. Others find periodic therapy helps maintain stability. Still others need ongoing support. All approaches are valid.

Signs therapy might help even if "fine":

- Life feels harder than it should
- Success requires enormous effort
- Relationships lack depth
- Work exhausts you completely
- Daily tasks feel overwhelming
- You're curious about easier ways

There's no shame in seeking support when functioning. Many autistic adults discover that "fine" was actually struggling, and support transforms their quality of life dramatically.

Key Takeaways

- Finding autism-informed healthcare providers requires strategic searching, careful vetting, and sometimes provider education
- Traditional therapy approaches need adaptation for autistic processing, sensory needs, and communication styles
- Occupational therapy offers practical support for daily living challenges often overlooked in adult services
- Co-occurring conditions are common and require integrated treatment considering autism's impact
- Medication management often requires adjusted dosing, careful monitoring, and consideration of sensory sensitivities
- Therapy benefits extend beyond crisis management to building sustainable life strategies
- Healthcare self-advocacy skills develop with practice and transform medical experiences

Building Daily Living Skills

Healthcare provides one foundation for wellbeing, but daily life management creates the structure for thriving. The next chapter explores practical strategies for managing executive function, sensory needs, and energy sustainably while preventing autistic burnout.

Chapter 10: Daily Living Strategies

Morning sunlight filters through carefully selected curtains—not too bright, not too dim. The coffee maker, programmed the night before, fills the kitchen with predictable aroma. Every item in the apartment has its designated place, each routine choreographed to minimize decision fatigue. This isn't obsessive behavior—it's an autistic adult creating an environment that works with their neurology. This chapter provides practical strategies for building sustainable daily living systems that honor your autistic needs.

Executive Function Supports

Executive function challenges affect most autistic adults, impacting everything from morning routines to major life decisions. Rather than fighting these differences, effective strategies work with your brain's natural patterns.

Understanding Your Executive Function Profile:

Executive function isn't monolithic—it includes multiple components that vary independently:

- **Working Memory**: Holding information while using it
- **Task Initiation**: Starting activities independently
- **Planning/Prioritization**: Organizing approach to tasks
- **Organization**: Managing materials and information
- **Time Management**: Sensing and allocating time
- **Goal-Directed Persistence**: Maintaining effort
- **Flexibility**: Adjusting to changes
- **Metacognition**: Self-monitoring and evaluation

Map your specific profile. You might excel at organization while struggling with task initiation, or manage time well but lack flexibility.

External Brain Systems:

Since executive function challenges are neurological, not character flaws, external supports become assistive technology:

Digital Systems:

- Calendar apps with multiple alerts
- Task management apps (Todoist, Notion, Trello)
- Time-tracking tools showing where time goes
- Automated bill payment and reminders
- Voice assistants for immediate capture
- Location-based reminders

Marcus created what he calls his "external executive function suite." His phone provides hourly chimes for time awareness. Location-based reminders alert him to buy groceries when near the store. His smartwatch taps for transition warnings. Voice commands capture thoughts immediately. This digital scaffolding replaced constant anxiety with reliable support.

Physical Systems:

- Launch pads by doors with needed items
- Visual schedules on walls
- Color-coded organization systems
- Timer cubes for time awareness
- Checklist templates for routines
- Bins labeled with photos

Routine as Executive Function Support:

Routines reduce executive function demands by automating decisions:

Morning Routine Example:

1. Alarm at consistent time
2. Bathroom routine (same order daily)
3. Breakfast (same 2-3 options rotating)
4. Dressing (pre-selected outfits)
5. Review day's schedule
6. Launch pad check
7. Leave at set time

Each step cues the next, eliminating decision points. When routines become automatic, executive function reserves remain for unexpected challenges.

Task Initiation Strategies:

Starting tasks often poses the biggest challenge:

- **Environmental cues**: Designate spaces for specific activities
- **Transition rituals**: Use stimming to shift between tasks
- **Minimum viable starts**: "Just open the document"
- **Body doubling**: Work alongside others (virtually or in-person)
- **Interest linking**: Connect tasks to special interests
- **External accountability**: Tell someone your intention

Jennifer struggled with work-from-home task initiation until developing her "activation sequence." She lights a specific candle, plays particular background music, and spends two minutes with her fidget cube. This ritual signals her brain to transition into work mode, bypassing the initiation struggle.

Planning and Prioritization Tools:

Transform abstract planning into concrete steps:

1. **Brain dumps**: List everything without organizing

2. **Categorization**: Sort by context, urgency, energy required
3. **Must/Should/Could framework**: Realistic prioritization
4. **Time-boxing**: Assign specific time blocks
5. **Buffer building**: Add 50% more time than estimated
6. **Review cycles**: Regular system evaluation

Sensory Management Techniques

Sensory differences profoundly impact daily living. Creating sensory-supportive environments and developing regulation strategies transforms quality of life.

Sensory Profiling:

Map your sensory needs across all eight senses:

Visual:

- Light sensitivity levels
- Color preferences/aversions
- Pattern tolerance
- Movement sensitivity
- Optimal lighting types

Auditory:

- Sound sensitivity patterns
- Helpful vs. harmful frequencies
- Background noise needs
- Voice/music preferences
- Silence requirements

Tactile:

- Texture preferences/aversions
- Pressure needs

- Temperature sensitivity
- Clothing requirements
- Touch boundaries

Gustatory/Olfactory:

- Taste sensitivities
- Texture issues
- Smell triggers
- Safe foods
- Environmental scents

Vestibular/Proprioceptive:

- Movement needs
- Balance challenges
- Body awareness
- Pressure preferences
- Spatial requirements

Interoceptive:

- Hunger/thirst awareness
- Pain perception
- Emotional body signals
- bathroom needs recognition
- Temperature regulation

David's sensory profile revealed seemingly contradictory needs—he craves deep pressure but can't tolerate light touch. Understanding this paradox let him seek weighted blankets while maintaining touch boundaries, significantly improving sleep and relationships.

Creating Sensory Sanctuaries:

Designate spaces for sensory regulation:

Bedroom Optimization:

- Blackout curtains or specific lighting
- White noise machine or silence
- Weighted blankets or light covers
- Temperature control
- Texture-appropriate bedding
- Minimal visual clutter

Regulation Station: Create a dedicated sensory space:

- Comfortable seating options
- Fidget tool collection
- Noise-canceling headphones
- Soft lighting options
- Temperature regulation tools
- Pleasant scents or air purifier

Portable Sensory Kits:

Build kits for different contexts:

Work Kit:

- Discrete fidgets
- Noise-reducing earplugs
- Sunglasses for fluorescents
- Preferred snacks
- Essential oil roller
- Stress ball

Travel Kit:

- Familiar pillowcase
- Travel white noise
- Comfort objects
- Safe foods

- Entertainment options
- Medical information

Daily Sensory Regulation:

Build regulation into daily routines:

Morning Regulation:

- Gradual light exposure
- Specific shower temperature/pressure
- Predictable breakfast textures
- Movement or stretching
- Preferred morning sounds

Workday Breaks:

- Scheduled regulation times
- Movement breaks
- Sensory snacks
- Quiet moments
- Deep pressure activities

Evening Wind-Down:

- Dimming lights gradually
- Calming activities
- Consistent bedtime routine
- Sensory preparation for sleep
- Review and reset space

Lisa schedules "sensory appointments" with herself—non-negotiable regulation times. Every two hours, she spends ten minutes with noise-canceling headphones, compression vest, and lavender scent. These preventive breaks prevent sensory overload accumulation.

Energy Management and Burnout Prevention

Autistic burnout—the state of complete physical, emotional, and cognitive exhaustion from cumulative life demands—affects most autistic adults. Prevention requires understanding your energy patterns and building sustainable systems (42).

Understanding Energy Economics:

Autistic adults often operate with different energy economics than neurotypicals:

- **Baseline energy costs**: Daily life requires more energy
- **Masking drain**: Social camouflaging depletes reserves
- **Sensory processing load**: Constant filtering exhausts
- **Executive function demands**: Each decision costs energy
- **Recovery needs**: Longer recuperation required

Think of energy as currency with finite daily allowance. Every activity has a cost:

- Video call: 50 energy units
- Grocery shopping: 75 units
- Masking at work: 200 units
- Special interest time: +30 units
- Sensory overload: -100 units

Identifying Burnout Warning Signs:

Early warning signs precede full burnout:

Cognitive Signs:

- Increased word-finding difficulty
- Executive function deterioration
- Decision paralysis over simple choices

- Memory lapses
- Processing delays

Physical Signs:

- Increased sensory sensitivity
- Sleep disruption
- Appetite changes
- Increased stimming
- Coordination changes

Emotional Signs:

- Irritability spike
- Emotional numbness
- Increased meltdowns/shutdowns
- Social withdrawal
- Loss of joy in interests

Behavioral Signs:

- Routine disruption
- Hygiene challenges
- Communication reduction
- Isolation increase
- Skill regression

Michael tracks his burnout indicators in a simple app, rating five key areas daily. When three indicators reach "yellow zone," he implements his "pressure release protocol"—canceling optional commitments, increasing alone time, and focusing on restoration.

Building Sustainable Schedules:

Prevention requires realistic scheduling:

1. **Energy budgeting**: Calculate activity costs realistically
2. **Recovery building**: Schedule restoration time
3. **Batch similar tasks**: Reduce transition costs
4. **Protect prime time**: Use best energy for priorities
5. **Buffer creation**: Allow 30-50% extra time
6. **Flexibility planning**: Build in adjustment space

The Sustainable Week Framework:

Design weeks balancing demands with restoration:

- **Monday**: Gentle start, routine tasks
- **Tuesday-Thursday**: Higher demand tolerance
- **Friday**: Wrap-up, lower demands
- **Weekend**: At least one full recovery day

Recovery Strategies:

Active recovery accelerates restoration:

Sensory Recovery:

- Complete silence or preferred sounds
- Darkness or specific lighting
- Comfortable temperature
- Preferred textures
- Movement or stillness

Cognitive Recovery:

- Special interest immersion
- Minimal decision-making
- Routine activities only
- No new information
- Creative expression

Social Recovery:

- Solitude or safe people only
- No masking requirements
- Written communication only
- Boundary enforcement
- Energy vampire avoidance

Physical Recovery:

- Adequate sleep
- Nutritious safe foods
- Gentle movement
- Hydration focus
- Medication consistency

Home Environment Modifications

Your living space significantly impacts daily functioning. Creating an autism-friendly home environment supports regulation, reduces stress, and enables thriving.

Organizational Systems:

Visual Organization:

- Clear containers showing contents
- Labels with words and pictures
- Color-coding systems
- Designated spots for everything
- Open shelving for easy access
- Minimal visual clutter

Functional Zones: Create specific areas for different activities:

- Work zone with needed supplies
- Relaxation area with comfort items
- Eating space with minimal distractions
- Sleep zone optimized for rest

- Movement/stimming space
- Quiet regulation corner

Sarah restructured her apartment into functional zones. Her "work pod" contains everything needed for remote work. The "restoration nook" holds weighted blankets, fidgets, and noise machine. Clear boundaries between zones help her brain transition between activities.

Lighting Solutions:

Lighting profoundly affects autistic wellbeing:

- **Natural light management**: Adjustable curtains/blinds
- **Artificial options**: Warm LED bulbs, salt lamps
- **Dimmer switches**: Control intensity
- **Task lighting**: Focused illumination
- **Color options**: Some prefer colored bulbs
- **Elimination**: Remove fluorescent fixtures

Sound Management:

Control auditory environment:

- **White noise machines**: Mask unpredictable sounds
- **Sound absorption**: Rugs, curtains, wall hangings
- **Noise isolation**: Weather stripping, door sweeps
- **Dedicated quiet spaces**: Sound-proofed areas
- **Nature sounds**: Calming background options

Temperature and Air Quality:

- **Consistent temperature**: Programmable thermostat
- **Air purification**: Remove irritating particles
- **Humidity control**: Optimal comfort levels
- **Fresh air access**: Windows or ventilation
- **Scent management**: Fragrance-free products

Safety Modifications:

Prevent injury during overload:

- **Soft corners**: Padding on sharp edges
- **Non-slip surfaces**: Reduce fall risk
- **Clear pathways**: Minimize obstacles
- **Emergency supplies**: Easily accessible
- **Comfort items**: Throughout space

Technology Tools and Apps

Technology offers powerful support for autistic daily living. The key lies in finding tools that genuinely help rather than adding complexity.

Communication Apps:

AAC Options:

- Proloquo2Go for comprehensive AAC
- Emergency Chat for temporary speech loss
- Card Talk for simple communication
- Text-to-speech options
- Symbol-based systems

Social Scripts:

- Conversation planning apps
- Email templates
- Social story creators
- Video modeling tools
- Practice scenarios

Executive Function Apps:

Time Management:

- Visual timers (Time Timer)
- Pomodoro apps with customization
- Calendar apps with multiple alerts
- Time tracking tools (Toggl, RescueTime)
- Routine apps (Routinery, Productive)

Task Management:

- Simple lists (Google Keep, Apple Notes)
- Project management (Notion, Asana)
- Habit tracking (Habitica, Streaks)
- Mind mapping (SimpleMind, MindMeister)
- Decision-making aids

Robert uses a combination of apps creating his "digital support team." Routinery guides morning routines with timed steps. Todoist breaks projects into tiny tasks. Forest app prevents phone distraction during focus time. Together, they compensate for executive function challenges.

Sensory Support Apps:

- **Sound generation**: White noise, nature sounds, binaural beats
- **Visual calm**: Lava lamp apps, pattern generators
- **Breathing guides**: Anxiety reduction tools
- **Movement reminders**: Stretch and regulation prompts
- **Sensory tracking**: Monitor triggers and patterns

Daily Living Apps:

Meal Planning:

- Apps accounting for sensory preferences
- Visual meal prep guides
- Grocery list generators
- Safe food trackers

- Nutrition monitoring

Financial Management:

- Automated bill pay
- Spending trackers with alerts
- Visual budget apps
- Subscription managers
- Receipt organizers

Health Tracking:

- Medication reminders
- Symptom tracking
- Sleep monitoring
- Appointment scheduling
- Emergency information

Choosing and Implementing Tools:

1. **Start small**: One app at a time
2. **Test thoroughly**: Use trial periods
3. **Customize extensively**: Adjust all settings
4. **Create backups**: Don't rely on single tool
5. **Regular reviews**: Evaluate effectiveness
6. **Permission to quit**: Not every tool works

FAQ: "How do I prevent autistic burnout?"

Preventing autistic burnout requires proactive strategies rather than reactive crisis management. Think of it like maintaining a car—regular maintenance prevents breakdowns.

Recognize Your Patterns:

Track your burnout cycles:

- What triggers overwhelm?
- How long between burnouts?
- Which warning signs appear first?
- What helps recovery?
- Which situations always drain you?

Build Prevention Systems:

Energy Management:

- Track energy income and expenses
- Schedule regular recharge time
- Protect energy reserves fiercely
- Say no to energy vampires
- Build restoration into daily life

Boundary Setting:

- Define non-negotiable needs
- Communicate limits clearly
- Practice boundary phrases
- Accept others' reactions
- Maintain boundaries consistently

Support Network Development:

- Identify safe people
- Build reciprocal relationships
- Ask for help early
- Create emergency plans
- Maintain connections sustainably

Emma prevents burnout through what she calls "aggressive self-care." She schedules two daily "power hours" for special interests. Wednesdays are "no people days." She tracks energy levels in a simple app, adjusting commitments when reserves drop. This proactive approach extended her between-burnout period from three months to over a year.

Lifestyle Design for Prevention:

- **Work**: Choose sustainable employment or modify current role
- **Home**: Create restorative environment
- **Relationships**: Surround yourself with understanding people
- **Activities**: Balance obligations with restoration
- **Health**: Maintain physical wellness foundations

Emergency Planning:

Despite prevention, prepare for burnout:

1. Document early warning signs
2. Create communication templates
3. Prepare easy meals/systems
4. Identify minimum obligations
5. Build recovery protocols
6. Share plan with support people

Burnout isn't failure—it's a sign that life demands exceed resources. Prevention means designing life within your sustainable capacity rather than constantly pushing limits. This might mean choices others don't understand, but your wellbeing matters more than meeting neurotypical expectations.

Key Takeaways

- Executive function supports through external systems, routines, and tools compensate for neurological differences
- Sensory management requires understanding your profile and creating supportive environments

- Energy management and burnout prevention demand proactive planning and sustainable scheduling
- Home environment modifications significantly impact daily functioning and wellbeing
- Technology tools offer powerful support when carefully selected and implemented
- Preventing burnout requires lifestyle design within your capacity rather than pushing through
- Daily living strategies work best when customized to your specific needs and preferences

Creating sustainable daily living systems provides the foundation for everything else—relationships, work, education, and personal growth. These strategies aren't about becoming more neurotypical but about building a life that works with your autistic neurology. As you implement these approaches, remember that small changes accumulate into profound transformation. Your daily life can shift from constant struggle to sustainable rhythm when you stop fighting your neurology and start supporting it.

Chapter 11: Relationships and Communication

The conversation replays in your mind for the hundredth time. Did your tone sound too flat? Was your explanation too detailed? Why did they look confused when you answered their question literally? For autistic adults, relationships often feel like performing in a play where everyone else has the script. This chapter provides practical strategies for building authentic connections, communicating your needs effectively, and maintaining relationships that honor your autistic identity.

Explaining Autism to Family and Friends

Sharing your autism diagnosis with loved ones can transform relationships—or complicate them. Each disclosure requires careful consideration of the person, your relationship dynamics, and your communication goals.

Understanding Different Reactions

Family and friends respond to autism disclosure in patterns you can anticipate and prepare for:

The Dismissers: "But you've always been like this!" or "Everyone's a little autistic." These responses often come from discomfort with change or misunderstanding autism. They're trying to maintain the status quo rather than acknowledging your reality.

The Researchers: Immediately googling everything about autism, sometimes becoming instant "experts." While their enthusiasm might feel overwhelming, it usually comes from caring and wanting to understand.

The Grievers: Acting as if you've shared tragic news. They're mourning their incorrect assumptions about your future or capabilities, not realizing autism isn't a tragedy.

The Supporters: "Thank you for trusting me. How can I support you?" These gems validate your experience and focus on your needs rather than their reactions.

Maria's family disclosure illustrates these varied responses. Her mother immediately dismissed it: "You graduated college—you can't be autistic." Her brother became a researcher, sending daily articles about autism "cures." Her sister grieved, crying about Maria's "difficult life ahead." Only her cousin responded supportively, asking how to make family gatherings more comfortable. Preparing for these reactions helped Maria stay centered despite the emotional chaos.

Crafting Your Explanation

Effective explanations balance education with personal experience:

Start with the personal: "I recently learned I'm autistic. This explains so many of my experiences..."

Address misconceptions directly: "Autism isn't just what you see in movies. For me, it means..."

Use concrete examples: "You know how I always need the plan for gatherings? That's because..."

Focus on positives too: "My attention to detail that helps me catch errors? That's part of being autistic."

Set boundaries: "I'm sharing this because I trust you, not asking for advice or fixes."

Preparation Strategies

Before disclosing:

1. **Choose your medium**: Face-to-face, phone, letter, or email?
2. **Pick optimal timing**: Not during stress or major events
3. **Prepare resources**: Have articles or books ready to share
4. **Practice key points**: Write out main messages
5. **Plan self-care**: Schedule recovery time afterward
6. **Consider partial disclosure**: Share with one person at a time

David wrote individual letters to family members, tailoring each to the relationship. His letter to his engineer father emphasized autism's pattern-recognition aspects. His artistic mother's letter discussed sensory experiences. His teenage nephew's email used gaming metaphors. This personalized approach helped each person understand autism through their own lens.

Managing Ongoing Conversations

Initial disclosure often begins ongoing dialogue:

- **Education takes time**: People need multiple conversations to understand
- **Model boundaries**: Show them how to respect your needs
- **Correct gently**: Address misconceptions without attacking
- **Share selectively**: You control how much detail to provide
- **Request specific support**: Tell them exactly how to help

Dating and Romantic Relationships

Romance adds layers of complexity to autistic communication. Building intimate relationships requires vulnerability about your needs while navigating neurotypical dating expectations.

Disclosure Timing in Dating

When to disclose remains individually determined:

Early disclosure (first few dates):

- Filters out incompatible people quickly
- Allows authentic presentation from start
- Reduces masking exhaustion
- May trigger prejudice before connection forms

Middle disclosure (after connection established):

- Person knows you beyond stereotypes
- Trust exists for vulnerable conversation
- Risk of feeling deceived about "hiding"
- Allows informed relationship decisions

Late disclosure (committed relationship):

- Maximum connection before revelation
- Highest risk of partner feeling betrayed
- May explain past relationship conflicts
- Requires significant trust rebuilding

Jennifer tried all three approaches across different relationships. Early disclosure led to immediate ghosting but saved energy. Middle disclosure worked best—partners knew her personality before processing autism information. Late disclosure in one relationship created trust issues that never fully healed. She now discloses around date four or five, after initial connection but before deep attachment.

Communication in Romantic Relationships

Autistic-neurotypical relationships require intentional communication strategies:

Direct communication preferences:

- "I need you to say exactly what you mean"
- "I won't pick up hints—please be direct"
- "When you say 'fine,' I believe you're fine"
- "I show love through actions, not words"

Sensory considerations:

- Discuss touch preferences explicitly
- Negotiate physical intimacy needs
- Plan sensory-friendly date activities
- Create intimate spaces respecting sensory needs

Emotional processing differences:

- "I need time to process emotions before discussing"
- "My flat expression doesn't mean I don't care"
- "I experience emotions intensely but express them differently"
- "Written communication helps me express feelings"

Practical strategies for relationship success:

1. **Regular relationship check-ins**: Scheduled conversations about needs
2. **Written communication**: Texts or emails for difficult topics
3. **Explicit expectations**: Clear discussion of relationship rules
4. **Parallel activities**: Being together without direct interaction

5. **Escape plans**: Agreement about leaving overwhelming situations

Michael and his neurotypical wife Sarah developed their "relationship operating manual" over five years. It includes his need for thirty minutes of silence after work, her need for daily verbal affection, their agreement about party exit strategies, and scripts for common conflicts. This explicit framework replaced assumptions with understanding.

Autistic-Autistic Relationships

Relationships between autistic partners offer unique advantages and challenges:

Advantages:

- Mutual understanding of sensory needs
- Direct communication appreciation
- Shared experience of navigating neurotypical world
- Less masking required
- Special interest sharing potential

Challenges:

- Conflicting sensory needs
- Executive function struggles multiplied
- Different communication styles within autism
- Competing routine requirements
- Limited social energy for relationship work

Lisa and Jamie, both autistic, created systems honoring their needs. They live in separate bedrooms for sensory control. Sunday mornings are parallel special interest time. They use shared calendars religiously. Their relationship thrives because they explicitly designed it around autistic needs rather than neurotypical relationship templates.

Parenting as an Autistic Adult

Autistic parents face unique challenges and possess distinct strengths. Understanding how autism affects parenting helps create family systems that work for everyone.

Autistic Parenting Strengths:

- **Consistency**: Routine-loving parents create predictable environments
- **Acceptance**: Understanding of children's differences
- **Logic**: Clear, rational explanations for rules
- **Special interests**: Deep engagement in children's interests
- **Sensory awareness**: Recognition of children's sensory needs
- **Direct communication**: No confusing mixed messages

Common Challenges:

Sensory overload from children: Children create constant sensory input—crying, unexpected touches, messes, noise. Managing parental overload while meeting children's needs requires strategy.

Executive function demands: Parenting involves constant planning, multitasking, and flexibility—all executive function challenges.

Social navigation: School events, playdates, and parent social expectations drain social energy.

Communication with co-parents: Different parenting styles between autistic and neurotypical parents need negotiation.

Rachel, autistic mother of two, structures parenting around her needs. Morning routines run like clockwork, reducing decision fatigue. She wears noise-reducing earplugs while maintaining safety awareness. Her "quiet hour" after school allows her recovery before homework time. Her children understand "Mommy needs quiet time" as normal family functioning.

Strategies for Sustainable Parenting:

1. **Build predictable routines**: Benefits both autistic parents and children
2. **Create sensory retreats**: Designated parent quiet spaces
3. **Use visual schedules**: For whole family organization
4. **Delegate overwhelming tasks**: Trade duties with co-parent or support system
5. **Model self-regulation**: Show children healthy coping strategies
6. **Prepare scripts**: For common parenting scenarios
7. **Build support networks**: Other parents who understand

Parenting Autistic Children:

Autistic parents of autistic children face specific considerations:

- **Genetic understanding**: Recognizing autism signs others might miss
- **Accommodation modeling**: Showing children self-advocacy
- **Avoiding projection**: Children's autism differs from yours
- **Double accommodation needs**: Managing multiple sensory profiles
- **Identity support**: Helping children develop positive autistic identity

Tom discovered his own autism through his son's diagnosis. Now he parents with deep understanding of his son's experiences while recognizing their different support needs. His son seeks sensory input; Tom avoids it. They've created family rules honoring both needs—trampolines in the basement for son, noise-canceling headphones for dad.

Friendship Maintenance Strategies

Adult friendships challenge autistic people differently than childhood connections. Without school's built-in structure, maintaining friendships requires intentional effort and systems.

Understanding Autistic Friendship Patterns:

- **Quality over quantity**: Few deep friendships rather than many acquaintances
- **Interest-based connections**: Bonding through shared activities
- **Parallel presence**: Being together without constant interaction
- **Inconsistent contact**: Intense connection periods followed by gaps
- **Loyalty depth**: Strong commitment once trust established

Common Friendship Challenges:

Initiation difficulties: Starting friendships without structured environments **Maintenance energy**: Remembering to reach out regularly **Reciprocity confusion**: Understanding unwritten friendship rules **Conflict navigation**: Direct communication misunderstood as rudeness **Social energy limits**: Balancing friendship needs with recovery time

Building Sustainable Friendships:

1. **Seek interest-aligned people**: Join clubs or groups around special interests
2. **Be explicit about needs**: "I care about you but need communication breaks"

3. **Create friendship routines**: Weekly game nights, monthly coffee dates
4. **Use technology**: Maintain connection through texts or online games
5. **Quality time planning**: Shorter, meaningful interactions over long social events

Anna maintains three close friendships through careful planning. Tuesday online gaming with Marcus, Saturday morning walks with Jennifer, and monthly book discussions with David. These structured interactions provide connection without overwhelming her social capacity. Friends understand her communication style and energy limits.

Scripts for Common Friendship Scenarios:

Explaining communication patterns: "I might not text for weeks, but it doesn't mean I don't care. My brain just doesn't prompt social reaching out."

Setting social boundaries: "I value our friendship and want to spend quality time together. I can do coffee for an hour but not all-day activities."

Addressing conflicts: "I think we had a misunderstanding. Can you tell me directly what upset you so I can understand?"

Setting Boundaries

Boundaries protect autistic adults from burnout while maintaining healthy relationships. Clear boundaries aren't selfishness—they're self-preservation.

Types of Boundaries Autistic Adults Need:

Sensory boundaries:

- "Please don't wear strong perfume around me"
- "I need advance warning before physical touch"
- "I can't eat at restaurants with fluorescent lighting"

Communication boundaries:

- "I prefer text over phone calls"
- "I need 24 hours to process before discussing emotional topics"
- "Please be direct rather than hinting"

Time and energy boundaries:

- "I can attend for one hour maximum"
- "I need one full day of recovery after social events"
- "Spontaneous plans don't work for me"

Space boundaries:

- "I need alone time daily"
- "Please knock before entering my space"
- "I can't share beds, even with partners"

Boundary Setting Process:

1. **Identify your needs**: What depletes you? What restores you?
2. **Practice stating boundaries**: Write scripts and rehearse
3. **Start small**: Set one boundary at a time
4. **Expect pushback**: People resist change initially
5. **Stay consistent**: Inconsistent enforcement creates confusion
6. **Offer alternatives**: "I can't do X, but I can do Y"

Mark learned boundary setting through painful trial. After years of burnout from saying yes to everything, he developed his "boundary toolkit." He now declines evening events, limits weekend socializing to one activity, and takes communication breaks. Initially, friends resisted. Some relationships ended. But remaining friendships became stronger and more authentic.

Maintaining Boundaries Against Pressure:

Common pressures and responses:

"Just this once": "My needs don't have exceptions. Let's find another solution."

"You're being difficult": "I'm being clear about my needs to maintain our relationship."

"You didn't used to be like this": "I've learned to advocate for my needs better."

"If you really cared...": "Caring means being honest about my limitations."

Chapter FAQ: "How do I explain my needs to my partner?"

Explaining your needs requires clarity, patience, and practical strategies. Your partner wants to understand but might need concrete guidance.

Start with education: Share resources about autism in relationships. Avoid overwhelming them—one article or video at a time. Choose materials reflecting your specific presentation.

Use concrete examples: Instead of "I have sensory issues," say "Fluorescent lights at the grocery store cause headaches. I need to shop at less busy times or wear sunglasses."

Connect needs to behaviors: "When I rock or fidget, I'm regulating my nervous system, not displaying anxiety about our relationship."

Create reference documents: Write guides about your needs:

- Sensory triggers and accommodations
- Communication preferences
- Emotional expression differences
- Energy management needs
- Meltdown/shutdown protocols

Regular check-ins: Schedule monthly relationship meetings to discuss what's working and what needs adjustment. Written agendas help structure these conversations.

Acknowledge their needs too: Relationships require mutual accommodation. Ask about their needs and collaborate on solutions honoring both perspectives.

Be patient with the process: Understanding develops over time. Celebrate small victories. One couple took two years to fully develop communication patterns that worked. Your partner's willingness to learn matters more than immediate perfection.

Susan created what she calls her "User Manual"—a document explaining her autistic traits and needs. It includes sections on communication ("I process literally—sarcasm confuses me"), sensory needs ("Please warn me before turning on the blender"), and emotional expression ("I show love through acts of service, not verbal affirmations"). Her partner references it regularly and they update it together as they learn.

The key is making your needs concrete and actionable rather than abstract concepts. Your partner can't accommodate needs they don't understand. Clear, specific communication creates the foundation for lasting relationship success.

Key Takeaways

- Explaining autism to family and friends requires preparation for varied reactions and ongoing education
- Dating and romantic relationships benefit from strategic disclosure timing and explicit communication
- Autistic parents can build family systems honoring their needs while nurturing children effectively
- Friendship maintenance requires intentional strategies and energy management
- Clear boundaries protect against burnout and enable sustainable relationships
- Partners need concrete, specific information to understand and accommodate autistic needs
- All relationships improve with direct communication and mutual respect for differences

Building Community Connections

Individual relationships form the foundation, but community provides broader support and understanding. The next chapter explores finding your people—other autistic adults who share your experiences and can offer wisdom from their own journeys. Together, we're stronger than alone.

Chapter 12: Finding Your Community

The relief feels almost physical when you first connect with other autistic adults. Suddenly, your experiences aren't strange or wrong—they're shared, understood, validated. That constant translation between your internal experience and external expression? Not needed here. Finding autistic community transforms isolation into belonging, confusion into clarity, and shame into pride. This chapter guides you through discovering, building, and nurturing the community connections that can change your life.

Online Autistic Communities

The internet revolutionized autistic community building. No longer limited by geography or social energy, autistic adults connect across distances, time zones, and communication preferences. Online spaces offer entry points for every comfort level and interest.

Major Platform Communities

Reddit Autism Communities:

- r/autism: General autism discussion
- r/AutismInWomen: Specific experiences of autistic women and femmes
- r/autisticadults: Adult-focused discussions
- r/aspergers: Active despite outdated terminology
- r/autisticpride: Neurodiversity-affirming space

Each subreddit has distinct culture. Read lurker-mode for weeks before participating. Notice communication styles, common topics, and community norms.

Facebook Groups: Private groups offer more intimate discussion. Search "[Your City] Autistic Adults" or interest-specific groups like "Autistic Parents" or "Autistic Professionals in Tech." Closed groups provide safety from public scrutiny.

Discord Servers: Real-time chat suits some autistic communication styles. Servers often organize channels by topic—sensory support, special interests, daily check-ins. Voice channels optional; most communication happens via text.

Twitter/X Communities: Hashtags like #ActuallyAutistic, #AutisticAdult, and #AskingAutistics connect community members. The platform's character limit can help concise communication. Block liberally to maintain positive space.

Specialized Platforms:

- Wrong Planet: Long-running autism community forum
- Autistic Not Weird: Facebook community with active discussion
- The Thinking Person's Guide to Autism: Community focused on advocacy

Emma discovered online community during post-diagnosis identity crisis. Starting as silent observer in Facebook groups, she gradually recognized her experiences in others' posts. First commenting with simple validations, then sharing her own experiences, she built connections that became real friendships. Her closest friends now live across three continents, connected through daily Discord chats about everything from special interests to sensory struggles.

Online Community Benefits:

- **24/7 availability**: Support when you need it
- **Asynchronous communication**: Respond at your pace
- **Anonymity options**: Share without real-name exposure

- **Global perspectives**: Learn from diverse experiences
- **Interest-based connections**: Find your specific tribes
- **Low social energy cost**: Engage from comfort zone

Navigating Online Spaces Safely:

1. **Verify autistic-led spaces**: Avoid parent-led or organization-controlled groups
2. **Check moderation policies**: Good communities have active, autistic moderators
3. **Start slowly**: Observe before engaging
4. **Protect privacy**: Use pseudonyms if preferred
5. **Trust instincts**: Leave spaces that feel wrong
6. **Block freely**: Your mental health matters more than politeness

Finding Your Online Niche:

Within broader communities, seek specific connections:

- Professional groups for your field
- Special interest communities
- Identity intersections (LGBTQ+ autistics, BIPOC autistics)
- Life stage groups (newly diagnosed, parents, seniors)
- Support-focused vs. social spaces

David found general autism groups overwhelming but thrived in "Autistic Software Engineers" Discord. The combination of shared neurology and profession created instant understanding. Members share coding tips adapted for autistic brains, discuss disclosure at tech companies, and celebrate pattern-recognition strengths in programming.

Local Support Groups

While online communities offer convenience, in-person connections provide unique benefits. Local groups create opportunities for masked adults to practice authenticity in safe spaces.

Finding Local Groups:

Search strategies:

- Autism organizations' directories (choose autistic-led when possible)
- Meetup.com autism or neurodiversity groups
- Library bulletin boards
- Disability resource centers
- University disability services
- Healthcare provider referrals
- Social media local searches

Types of Local Groups:

Support Groups: Traditional discussion-based meetings focusing on challenges and strategies. Usually facilitated, with structured sharing time.

Social Groups: Activity-based gatherings—board game nights, hiking groups, crafting circles. Parallel activities reduce direct social pressure.

Advocacy Groups: Focus on systemic change, disability rights, and community education. Channel frustration into action.

Professional Networks: Career-focused groups for workplace strategies and networking within neurological comfort zone.

Special Interest Groups: Not explicitly autistic but naturally attract autistic members—model train clubs, specialized book clubs, coding meetups.

Jennifer's journey illustrates local group evolution. Her city's single autism support group felt patronizing, run by non-autistic professionals. She connected with three other frustrated members. Together, they started "Actually Autistic [City Name]," meeting monthly at the library. Beginning with four members, they now host twenty regulars who've become genuine friends.

Making Groups Work for You:

Preparation strategies:

1. **Visit location beforehand**: Reduce arrival anxiety
2. **Contact facilitator**: Discuss accommodations needed
3. **Bring comfort items**: Fidgets, noise protection
4. **Plan exit strategy**: Know you can leave anytime
5. **Start small**: Attend briefly initially
6. **Decompress afterward**: Schedule recovery time

Group Meeting Accommodations:

Request what you need:

- Agenda provided in advance
- Lighting adjustments
- Break times
- Written communication options
- Fidget-friendly policy
- Fragrance-free space
- Clear time boundaries

Starting Your Own Group:

If nothing exists locally:

1. **Start tiny**: Even two people count

2. **Choose accessible locations**: Libraries, community centers
3. **Set clear boundaries**: Autistic-only spaces are valid
4. **Rotate facilitation**: Prevent burnout
5. **Keep it simple**: Conversation is enough
6. **Build slowly**: Growth takes time

Mark started "Autistic Coffee Hour" after finding no local options. Meeting Saturday mornings at a quiet café corner, the group began with him and one other person. Low-key format—show up, order coffee, chat or sit quietly—attracted members who found traditional support groups overwhelming. Two years later, fifteen regulars rotate between three café locations to accommodate sensory preferences.

Advocacy Organizations

Advocacy organizations offer structured ways to create change while building community. Choose carefully—many autism organizations aren't autistic-led.

Evaluating Organizations:

Green flags:

- Autistic leadership at all levels
- "Nothing about us without us" philosophy
- Neurodiversity paradigm adoption
- Focus on accommodation, not cure
- Amplifying autistic voices
- Intersectional approach

Red flags:

- Puzzle piece symbolism
- Cure-focused research
- Parent/professional leadership only

- ABA therapy promotion
- Functioning labels use
- Inspiration porn messaging

Major Autistic-Led Organizations:

Autistic Self Advocacy Network (ASAN): US-based but internationally influential. Focuses on policy change, community education, and resource development. Local chapters offer involvement opportunities.

Autistic Women & Nonbinary Network (AWN): Addresses gender-specific autistic experiences. Provides resources, advocacy, and community building.

Academic Autistic Spectrum Partnership in Research and Education (AASPIRE): Collaborative research including autistic adults as partners, not subjects.

Local Organizations: Many cities have grassroots autistic-led groups. Search "[city] autistic advocacy" or "[state] neurodiversity."

Sarah's advocacy journey began attending ASAN chapter meetings. Initially just listening, she gradually joined campaigns for employment rights. Working alongside other autistic advocates taught her more about autism than years of clinical literature. The shared purpose created bonds beyond typical social connections.

Ways to Engage:

Low-energy involvement:

- Sign petitions
- Share social media campaigns
- Donate if able

- Attend virtual events

Medium engagement:

- Join committees
- Write to legislators
- Participate in awareness campaigns
- Volunteer at events

High involvement:

- Board membership
- Leading campaigns
- Public speaking
- Media representation

Peer Mentorship Programs

Peer mentorship connects experienced autistic adults with those newer to diagnosis or seeking guidance. These relationships offer unique understanding impossible from neurotypical mentors.

Benefits of Autistic Mentors:

- **Lived experience wisdom**: Practical strategies that actually work
- **Identity development**: Models of thriving autistic adults
- **Communication ease**: Less translation needed
- **Validation**: Someone who truly "gets it"
- **Hope**: Proof that fulfilling life is possible

Finding Mentorship:

Formal Programs:

- Autism organizations often coordinate matching

- University disability services may offer programs
- Workplace neurodiversity initiatives
- Online mentorship platforms

Informal Connections:

- Reach out to autistic adults you admire
- Ask in online communities
- Connect at local meetings
- Build naturally from friendships

Being a Mentor:

Consider mentoring others when ready:

- Share your journey honestly
- Respect different support needs
- Avoid prescriptive advice
- Model self-advocacy
- Maintain boundaries

Robert found his mentor through an ASAN program. Marcus, diagnosed ten years earlier, guided Robert through workplace disclosure, sensory accommodation strategies, and relationship navigation. Weekly video calls provided consistent support. Marcus's acceptance of Robert's traits while sharing improvement strategies balanced validation with growth.

Mentorship Best Practices:

For Mentees:

1. Identify specific goals
2. Communicate preferred meeting structure
3. Respect mentor's time and energy
4. Apply suggestions before seeking more
5. Offer reciprocal support

For Mentors:

1. Share experiences, not rules
2. Acknowledge different presentations
3. Maintain confidentiality
4. Know your limits
5. Connect mentees to additional resources

Building Chosen Family

For many autistic adults, chosen family provides deeper understanding than biological relatives. These intentional relationships create support networks based on mutual choice rather than obligation.

Understanding Chosen Family:

Chosen family means:

- Intentional commitment to mutual support
- Acceptance without masking requirements
- Shared values and understanding
- Reciprocal care through challenges
- Celebration of authentic selves

Building Process:

Start with one: Deep connection with single person **Grow organically**: Let relationships develop naturally **Communicate explicitly**: Discuss chosen family intentions **Create rituals**: Regular gatherings or check-ins **Honor differences**: Autistic chosen family still has varying needs **Maintain flexibility**: Relationships ebb and flow

Lisa's chosen family emerged from her autism support group. Six members bonded deeply over two years. They formalized their connection, creating weekly dinners, emergency support protocols, and holiday traditions. When Lisa experienced autistic burnout, her chosen family provided meals, companionship, and advocacy with her employer—support her biological family couldn't understand to give.

Chosen Family Strategies:

1. **Regular gatherings**: Predictable connection times
2. **Communication agreements**: How to stay in touch
3. **Support protocols**: Plans for helping during crises
4. **Celebration traditions**: Honoring milestones together
5. **Conflict resolution**: Direct communication agreements
6. **Respecting autonomy**: Independence within connection

Virtual Chosen Family:

Online relationships can form chosen family:

- Daily check-ins through chat
- Virtual movie nights
- Parallel body doubling sessions
- Crisis support networks
- Celebration channels
- Long-term commitment

Alex's chosen family spans continents. Five autistic adults who met in Discord maintain daily connection through scheduled chats, memes sharing, and mutual support. They've supported each other through diagnoses, job losses, and relationship changes. Their commitment rivals any in-person family.

Chapter FAQ: "Where do I find other autistic adults?"

Finding autistic community requires multiple strategies since we don't have obvious gathering places. Start with these approaches:

Online First: Begin with online communities for low-pressure exploration:

- Search #ActuallyAutistic on social media
- Join platform-specific autism groups
- Participate in autism-focused Discord servers
- Follow autistic content creators
- Engage gradually as comfort allows

Local Searching:

- Contact disability resource centers
- Check library community boards
- Search Meetup for neurodiversity groups
- Ask healthcare providers for referrals
- Look for special interest groups that naturally attract autistics

Create Opportunities: If nothing exists, create it:

- Post in local online groups about meeting
- Start simple coffee meetups
- Organize around shared interests
- Keep initial expectations low
- Build consistency over time

Indirect Routes:

- LGBTQ+ spaces (high autistic overlap)
- Gaming communities
- Specialized hobby groups
- Academic environments
- Tech/STEM gatherings

Be Patient: Community building takes time. Many autistic adults isolate due to past rejection. Creating safe, consistent opportunities helps others feel secure engaging.

Daniel searched six months before finding community. Online groups felt overwhelming. Local autism organization was parent-focused. Finally, a librarian mentioned their unofficial "Quiet Crafts Hour" attracted many autistic adults. That weekly gathering became his entry point to local community.

Key is trying multiple avenues. What works varies by location, personality, and life circumstances. Keep searching—your people exist.

Key Takeaways

- Online communities offer 24/7 support with varied engagement levels and global connections
- Local support groups provide in-person practice being authentically autistic
- Choose advocacy organizations led by autistic people for authentic representation
- Peer mentorship offers guidance from lived experience perspective
- Chosen family creates intentional support networks beyond biological relations
- Finding community requires patience and multiple strategies
- Both online and offline connections serve different but important needs

Your Ongoing Journey

Community transforms the autistic experience from isolation to connection, from shame to pride. Finding your people—online, locally, or both—provides the foundation for thriving as your authentic autistic self. These connections offer more than support; they provide models for living, validation for your experiences, and hope for your future. You deserve community that celebrates rather than tolerates your autism. Keep searching until you find it.

Chapter 13: Reframing Your Past

The photo album sits open on your lap, each image now telling a different story. That birthday party where you hid under the table? Not defiance—sensory overload. The obsessive rock collection that drove your parents crazy? A special interest that brought order to chaos. Years of feeling fundamentally flawed suddenly shift into focus: you were never broken, just autistic in a world that didn't recognize it. This chapter guides you through the profound process of rewriting your personal history with compassion, understanding, and newfound clarity.

Understanding Your Life Through an Autistic Lens

Receiving an autism diagnosis in adulthood initiates a complete reexamination of your life story. Memories, struggles, and patterns that seemed random or character flaws suddenly form a coherent narrative. This reframing process can be simultaneously liberating and destabilizing.

The Reframing Process

Reframing involves examining past experiences through the filter of autism understanding:

Childhood Behaviors:

- "Difficult" becomes "overwhelmed"
- "Shy" becomes "socially anxious due to communication differences"
- "Picky eater" becomes "sensory food aversions"
- "Stubborn" becomes "needing predictability"
- "Dramatic" becomes "emotional dysregulation"

School Experiences:

- Academic success masking social struggles
- Friendlessness explained by different social needs
- Teacher complaints about "potential not met" reflecting executive function challenges
- Bullying targeting autistic traits
- Special interests dismissed as obsessions

Adult Patterns:

- Job hopping due to burnout, not laziness
- Relationship failures from communication differences
- Chronic health issues from sustained stress
- Mental health struggles from masking
- Life choices reflecting unconscious accommodations

Sarah spent months after diagnosis creating what she called her "autism autobiography." She reviewed old report cards with new eyes. "Sarah needs to participate more in group activities" transformed from personal failing to recognition of autistic social differences. Her third-grade teacher's note—"Sarah seems to live in her own world"—became evidence of rich inner life, not detachment. Each reframed memory helped rebuild her self-concept from "weird and wrong" to "autistic and misunderstood."

Common Reframing Revelations

Adults often recognize these patterns:

1. **Friendship struggles weren't personal failures**: Different social needs and communication styles created barriers
2. **Career difficulties reflected support needs**: Not lack of ability or motivation
3. **Sensory issues explained "pickiness"**: Food, clothing, and environment preferences were neurological needs

4. **Mental health issues had roots**: Depression and anxiety often stemmed from masking and overwhelm
5. **Coping mechanisms were adaptations**: What seemed like quirks were survival strategies

The Identity Shift

This reframing creates fundamental identity changes:

- From "lazy" to "executive function challenged"
- From "oversensitive" to "sensory processing differences"
- From "antisocial" to "needing social recovery"
- From "rigid" to "needing predictability"
- From "failed neurotypical" to "successful autistic"

Michael's reframing journey revealed decades of self-accommodation. His "hermit phase" in college? Burnout recovery. His obsession with routine? Anxiety management. His career in night-shift IT? Avoiding office social demands. Recognizing these as autism adaptations, not personality flaws, transformed his self-hatred into self-understanding.

Healing from Misdiagnosis and Trauma

Many late-diagnosed adults carry trauma from years of misunderstanding, misdiagnosis, and mistreatment. Healing requires acknowledging these wounds while building new, compassionate narratives.

Common Misdiagnoses

Before accurate autism diagnosis, many adults receive multiple incorrect labels:

- Anxiety disorders (without recognizing autism as root cause)
- Depression (from masking exhaustion)

- Borderline personality disorder (especially in women)
- Bipolar disorder (meltdowns mistaken for mood episodes)
- ADHD (though often co-occurs)
- Personality disorders
- Psychotic disorders (from describing sensory experiences)

Each misdiagnosis often came with inappropriate treatments—medications for wrong conditions, therapies targeting symptoms not causes, hospitalizations for autistic crises misread as psychiatric emergencies.

Jennifer's psychiatric history included seven diagnoses over fifteen years: major depression, generalized anxiety, social phobia, ADHD, borderline personality disorder, bipolar II, and avoidant personality disorder. Dozens of medications caused severe side effects without addressing core issues. CBT for social anxiety failed because her social struggles stemmed from communication differences, not distorted thinking. Only autism diagnosis at 38 finally explained the full picture. Previous diagnoses weren't entirely wrong—she did experience anxiety and depression—but they were effects, not causes.

Types of Autism-Related Trauma

Educational Trauma:

- Punishment for stimming or autistic behaviors
- Forced eye contact
- Public humiliation for social mistakes
- Bullying without protection
- Academic potential dismissed due to social differences

Medical Trauma:

- Invalidation of sensory experiences

- Forced compliance in overwhelming environments
- Mismedication effects
- Psychiatric hospitalizations for meltdowns
- Medical procedures without accommodation

Social Trauma:

- Repeated rejection without understanding why
- Manipulation by those who recognized vulnerability
- Constant correction of natural behaviors
- Isolation and loneliness
- Betrayal by trusted people

Family Trauma:

- Parents' frustration with "difficult" child
- Siblings' resentment of different needs
- Extended family's criticism
- Lack of protection from overwhelm
- Love conditional on appearing "normal"

David's trauma history included decades of educational abuse. Teachers physically stopped his rocking. Parents punished hand-flapping. Therapists tried to extinguish his special interests. ABA-style interventions taught him his natural ways of being were wrong. At 45, he works with a trauma-informed therapist to process these experiences, grieving the child who learned to hate his autistic self.

Healing Approaches

Recovery from autism-related trauma requires specialized approaches:

1. **Find autism-informed therapy**: Traditional therapy may retraumatize

2. **Process grief**: For support never received, life possibilities lost
3. **Anger validation**: Rage at systemic failures is justified
4. **Body-based healing**: Somatic approaches help stored trauma
5. **Community connection**: Others' similar experiences validate
6. **Narrative rewriting**: From victim to survivor to thriver

Celebrating Autistic Strengths

Amid processing difficulties, recognizing and celebrating autistic strengths proves essential for balanced identity development. Society focuses on autistic deficits, but our differences include powerful abilities.

Common Autistic Strengths

Pattern Recognition: Seeing connections others miss Many autistic adults excel in fields requiring pattern identification—data analysis, research, quality control, music, mathematics. This ability extends beyond professional applications to understanding complex systems intuitively.

Detail Perception: Noticing minute differences While others see forests, we see each tree's unique characteristics. This manifests in exceptional proofreading, artistic precision, scientific observation, and quality assessment.

Deep Focus: Sustained concentration on interests Hyperfocus enables mastery levels neurotypicals rarely achieve. Hours dissolve while engaged with fascinating topics, leading to expertise development.

Systematic Thinking: Understanding rule-based systems From computer programming to linguistics to legal frameworks, autistic minds often grasp systematic structures intuitively.

Honest Communication: Direct, truthful interaction Though sometimes socially penalized, autistic honesty creates trustworthy relationships and ethical decision-making.

Loyalty and Reliability: Deep commitment once trust established Autistic people often demonstrate fierce loyalty in relationships and reliability in responsibilities.

Creative Problem-Solving: Unique perspective generating novel solutions Thinking differently leads to innovative approaches others wouldn't consider.

Lisa discovered her autistic strengths through career analysis. Her "obsessive" attention to detail made her an exceptional editor. Her "inflexibility" about grammar rules meant catching errors others missed. Her "antisocial" preference for solo work meant deep focus producing high-quality output. Reframing weaknesses as profession-aligned strengths transformed her career satisfaction.

Strength Identification Exercise

Map your personal strengths:

1. List activities that feel effortless
2. Note compliments received repeatedly
3. Identify what others find difficult that seems easy
4. Consider special interest applications
5. Examine career successes
6. Ask trusted people about your abilities

Building on Strengths

Once identified, actively develop strengths:

- Seek roles utilizing natural abilities
- Stop forcing improvement in challenge areas

- Build confidence through strength application
- Share abilities with others
- Mentor in strength areas
- Create portfolio demonstrating abilities

Robert's strength mapping revealed unexpected patterns. His "weird" memory for conversations became valuable in legal work. His need for justice and rule-following made him exceptional at compliance. His pattern recognition caught financial irregularities. Building career around strengths rather than forcing neurotypical skills transformed professional success.

Letting Go of Shame

Shame runs deep for adults who spent decades believing they were fundamentally flawed. Releasing this shame requires conscious work and self-compassion.

Understanding Internalized Shame

Years of negative messages create internalized beliefs:

- "I'm too much" (from others' overwhelm at our intensity)
- "I'm not enough" (from failing neurotypical standards)
- "I'm broken" (from constant correction)
- "I'm unlovable" (from repeated rejection)
- "I'm lazy" (from executive function struggles)
- "I'm stupid" (from communication differences)

These beliefs formed when you lacked framework for understanding differences. They protected you by attempting to explain painful experiences but now limit growth.

Shame Release Strategies

Cognitive Restructuring: Challenge each shame-based belief:

- What evidence supports this?
- Would I say this to another autistic person?
- How does autism explain this differently?
- What would compassionate reframing sound like?

Somatic Release: Shame lives in the body:

- Notice where shame physically manifests
- Use movement to discharge stored emotion
- Try therapeutic shaking or dancing
- Practice self-soothing touch
- Engage in regulating sensory activities

Community Healing:

- Share shame stories with other autistic adults
- Witness others' similar experiences
- Receive validation and understanding
- Practice vulnerability in safe spaces
- Build new narratives together

Maria carried deep shame about meltdowns. Years of being called "dramatic," "attention-seeking," and "manipulative" created self-hatred. Through autistic community, she learned meltdowns are neurological events, not character flaws. Sharing meltdown experiences with others who understood began dissolving decades of shame. She now recognizes meltdowns as nervous system overload, responding with self-compassion rather than self-attack.

Self-Compassion Development

Replace shame with understanding:

1. Speak to yourself as beloved friend
2. Acknowledge past survival strategies
3. Honor child-you who did their best

4. Celebrate current growth
5. Practice daily self-forgiveness
6. Build self-compassion habits

Writing Your New Narrative

Creating new life story integrating autism understanding transforms identity from shame-based to strength-based. This narrative work provides foundation for future growth.

Elements of New Narrative

Honoring Survival: "I survived decades without support or understanding" **Recognizing Adaptations**: "I created innovative solutions to neurological differences" **Claiming Strengths**: "My autistic traits include valuable abilities" **Accepting Challenges**: "I have legitimate support needs" **Embracing Identity**: "I am autistic and worthwhile"

Narrative Writing Exercises

Timeline Revision: Create life timeline marking:

- Autistic traits emergence
- Adaptation strategies developed
- Burnout/crisis points
- Successes despite barriers
- Support that helped
- Current understanding

Letter Writing:

- To child-you explaining what was happening
- To past critics reframing their misunderstanding
- To current self offering compassion
- To future self describing hopes

Story Formats:

- Hero's journey with autism discovery as transformation
- Mystery solved by diagnosis revelation
- Adventure story of navigating neurotypical world
- Love story of self-acceptance

James wrote his narrative as science fiction—an alien descobering they'd been living among humans, explaining all miscommunications and cultural confusion. This metaphor helped him process experiences with humor and distance, reducing emotional overwhelm while building understanding.

Chapter FAQ: "How do I stop feeling broken?"

Feeling broken stems from decades of measuring yourself against neurotypical standards you could never meet. Healing requires fundamental perspective shift.

You're not broken—you're different. Autism means your neurology works differently, not wrongly. A Mac isn't a broken PC; it's a different operating system. You've spent years trying to run Windows software on Mac hardware. No wonder nothing worked right.

Practical steps to shift perspective:

1. **Language matters**: Notice self-talk using "broken," "wrong," "failed." Replace with "different," "challenged," "unsupported"
2. **Seek autistic perspectives**: Read autistic authors, follow autistic content creators, join autistic communities. Seeing successful autistic adults contradicts broken narratives
3. **Identify internalized ableism**: Question beliefs about productivity, social success, independence. Whose standards are these?

4. **Build on what works**: Focus energy on strengths and interests rather than fixing deficits
5. **Find your reference group**: Compare yourself to other autistic people, not neurotypical standards
6. **Practice radical acceptance**: You are exactly who you're supposed to be

Emily felt broken until finding autistic community online. Seeing others share her exact experiences—the social exhaustion, sensory overwhelm, communication struggles—shifted everything. She wasn't a failed neurotypical; she was a successful autistic person navigating an incompatible world. Her challenges weren't personal failures but systemic barriers.

Healing happens gradually. Some days, old "broken" feelings resurface. That's normal. Notice them, offer self-compassion, and return to truth: you were never broken, just misunderstood—most of all by yourself.

Key Takeaways

- Reframing past experiences through an autistic lens transforms self-understanding from "failed" to "unsupported"
- Healing from misdiagnosis and trauma requires specialized, autism-informed approaches
- Autistic strengths deserve recognition and celebration alongside challenge acknowledgment
- Releasing deep shame requires cognitive, somatic, and community-based healing
- Writing new personal narratives integrates autism understanding into identity
- Feeling broken stems from wrong standards, not personal failure
- Identity reconstruction is ongoing process requiring patience and self-compassion

Building Your Future

Understanding your past creates foundation for intentional future. No longer constrained by shame and misunderstanding, you can build life aligned with your authentic autistic self. The next chapter examines practical future planning—from daily sustainability to long-term security—designed around your actual needs rather than neurotypical assumptions.

Chapter 14: Future Planning

Your future stretches ahead, no longer constrained by impossibly neurotypical expectations. The diagnosis that explained your past now empowers you to build a future honoring your autistic needs. Gone are the days of forcing yourself into molds that never fit. This chapter provides practical frameworks for creating sustainable, fulfilling life plans that work with your neurology rather than against it.

Long-term Support Needs

Planning for long-term support requires honest assessment of your needs across life domains. Many autistic adults minimize support needs, having internalized ableist messages about independence. True independence means having support systems enabling you to thrive.

Assessing Support Needs Realistically

Support needs fluctuate across time and contexts. Map your needs across several dimensions:

Daily Living Support:

- Meal planning and preparation
- Household management
- Financial organization
- Healthcare coordination
- Transportation
- Personal care during burnout

Communication Support:

- Phone call assistance
- Written communication help

- Advocacy in meetings
- Social event navigation
- Conflict resolution
- Emergency communication plans

Executive Function Support:

- Schedule management
- Task prioritization
- Decision-making assistance
- Paperwork completion
- Deadline tracking
- System maintenance

Emotional/Social Support:

- Regular check-ins
- Crisis support protocols
- Social activity partners
- Isolation prevention
- Processing assistance
- Celebration sharing

Marcus thought he needed no support—he had a job, apartment, and car. But honest assessment revealed hidden struggles: eating the same three meals because meal planning overwhelmed him, avoiding medical care due to phone call anxiety, accumulating late fees from bill-paying executive dysfunction.
Acknowledging these needs allowed him to build supports: meal delivery service, online healthcare platforms, automatic bill pay. His life transformed from constant struggle to sustainable rhythm.

Types of Support Systems

Informal Support Networks:

- Family members (if supportive)
- Chosen family
- Friends and partners
- Online communities
- Neighbors
- Interest-based groups

Professional Support Services:

- Therapists and counselors
- Case managers
- Life coaches
- Professional organizers
- Assistive technology
- Home health aides

Community Resources:

- Disability service organizations
- Vocational rehabilitation
- Independent living centers
- Peer support programs
- Advocacy organizations
- Religious communities

Building Redundant Support

Single support sources create vulnerability. Build multiple layers:

1. **Primary supports**: Daily or frequent assistance
2. **Secondary supports**: Backup when primary unavailable
3. **Emergency supports**: Crisis intervention
4. **Professional supports**: Formal services
5. **Peer supports**: Others with lived experience
6. **Self-support tools**: Systems for independent functioning

Lisa's support web includes her partner (daily emotional support), autistic best friend (weekly check-ins), therapist (monthly sessions), online community (24/7 availability), meal kit service (nutrition support), and elaborate reminder systems (executive function support). When her partner travels, predetermined backup plans activate.

Financial Planning Considerations

Financial planning for autistic adults involves unique considerations around employment sustainability, support costs, and potential benefit eligibility.

Employment Sustainability Planning

Many autistic adults experience irregular employment due to:

- Burnout cycles requiring breaks
- Difficulty maintaining full-time work
- Need for specific work environments
- Communication challenges in traditional workplaces
- Sensory barriers to many jobs

Plan for employment variability:

- Build larger emergency funds (6-12 months expenses)
- Develop multiple income streams
- Consider part-time or flexible work
- Investigate remote opportunities
- Build skills enabling self-employment
- Maintain benefit eligibility if relevant

David structures finances around burnout cycles. After three job losses to autistic burnout, he built freelance graphic design business. Working from home eliminates sensory triggers. Flexible schedule accommodates energy fluctuations. He maintains nine-month expense buffer for inevitable burnout periods. This realistic planning reduced financial crisis stress.

Disability Benefits Navigation

Understanding disability benefit programs helps long-term planning:

Social Security Disability Insurance (SSDI):

- Based on work history
- No asset limits
- Can work part-time within limits
- Medicare eligibility after waiting period

Supplemental Security Income (SSI):

- Need-based program
- Strict asset limits
- Reduced by any income
- Medicaid eligibility included

ABLE Accounts:

- Tax-advantaged savings for disabled individuals
- Doesn't affect benefit eligibility
- Annual contribution limits
- Must be disabled before age 26

Many autistic adults struggle with benefit applications designed around visible disabilities. Document functional limitations thoroughly. Seek assistance from disability lawyers or advocates. Appeals are common—initial denials don't mean ineligibility.

Future Care Funding

Consider potential future support costs:

- Assisted living or supportive housing
- In-home support services
- Therapeutic services
- Assistive technology
- Transportation needs
- Healthcare costs

Funding strategies:

- Long-term care insurance (if obtainable)
- Special needs trusts
- ABLE accounts
- Health savings accounts
- Life insurance for caregivers
- Estate planning considerations

Healthcare Directives

Healthcare directives ensure your autistic needs are respected during medical crises when you cannot advocate for yourself.

Essential Healthcare Documents

Healthcare Proxy/Power of Attorney: Designate trusted person to make medical decisions. Choose someone who:

- Understands autism deeply
- Respects your autonomy
- Communicates effectively with providers
- Remains calm in crisis
- Knows your specific needs

Living Will/Advance Directives: Document treatment preferences including:

- Life-sustaining treatment wishes
- Pain management preferences
- Comfort care priorities
- Sensory accommodation needs
- Communication requirements

Hospital Autism Alert Card: Create card explaining:

- Autism diagnosis
- Communication needs
- Sensory sensitivities
- Behavioral responses to stress
- Helpful accommodations
- Emergency contact

Jennifer created comprehensive healthcare directives after a traumatic emergency room experience where staff misinterpreted autistic shutdown as psychiatric crisis. Her documents now clearly state: "Patient is autistic. During medical stress may become nonverbal, rock, or appear unresponsive. This is neurological, not psychiatric. Provide quiet environment, minimal questions, and written communication options." Her healthcare proxy carries detailed autism accommodation guide.

Autism-Specific Medical Planning

Include autism considerations:

Communication Plans:

- Nonverbal episode protocols
- AAC device instructions
- Processing time needs
- Literal interpretation notes
- Question simplification needs

Sensory Accommodations:

- Lighting preferences
- Sound sensitivity
- Touch precautions
- Medication sensitivities
- Environmental needs

Behavioral Explanations:

- Stimming descriptions
- Meltdown/shutdown appearance
- Stress responses
- Comfort objects
- Routine needs

Creating Provider Instructions

Develop one-page summary for medical providers:

- Autism diagnosis prominently displayed
- Communication methods
- Do's and don'ts list
- Sensory accommodations
- Medication sensitivities
- Emergency contact information

Building Sustainable Routines

Long-term success requires routines that support rather than constrain. Sustainable routines balance structure needs with flexibility for life's variations.

Elements of Sustainable Routines

Energy Management:

- High-energy tasks during peak times
- Low-demand activities when depleted

- Regular recharge periods
- Burnout prevention breaks
- Seasonal adjustments

Sensory Regulation:

- Morning sensory preparation
- Workday regulation breaks
- Evening wind-down sequences
- Weekend recovery time
- Crisis regulation protocols

Executive Function Supports:

- Consistent wake/sleep times
- Meal planning systems
- Task batching
- Decision reduction
- System maintenance time

Social Energy Balance:

- Scheduled social interactions
- Protected alone time
- Recovery after events
- Communication boundaries
- Relationship maintenance

Robert's routine evolution illustrates sustainability. Initial rigid schedule allowed no variation, leading to crisis when disrupted. Now his routine has flexibility built in: core morning sequence (shower, breakfast, review day) stays consistent, but afternoon varies by energy. Wednesday is always low-demand. Weekend mornings are unscheduled. This structure-with-flexibility maintains stability while preventing rigidity.

Routine Building Process

1. **Track natural patterns**: When do you have energy? Need rest?
2. **Identify non-negotiables**: What must happen for functioning?
3. **Build core structures**: Morning, evening, weekly anchors
4. **Add flexibility buffers**: Space for unexpected events
5. **Test and adjust**: Try for two weeks, then modify
6. **Regular reviews**: Quarterly routine assessments

Seasonal and Life Stage Adjustments

Routines must adapt to:

- Seasonal light/weather changes
- Age-related energy shifts
- Life circumstance changes
- Health status variations
- Support availability changes

Plan routine modifications for predictable changes. Sarah adjusts routines seasonally: summer's long light requires blackout curtains and earlier wind-down. Winter's darkness needs light therapy and vitamin D. Spring allergies require medication timing. Fall schedule changes need gradual transition. Anticipating adjustments prevents disruption.

Advocacy and Giving Back

Many late-diagnosed adults feel called to advocacy, wanting to ease the path for others. Sustainable advocacy requires balancing passion with capacity.

Forms of Advocacy

Personal Advocacy:

- Living openly autistic
- Educating friends/family
- Workplace accommodation modeling
- Social media presence
- Conversation participation

Community Advocacy:

- Support group facilitation
- Mentoring newly diagnosed
- Resource creation
- Story sharing
- Peer support provision

Systems Advocacy:

- Policy change work
- Organizational consulting
- Research participation
- Public speaking
- Media representation

Professional Advocacy:

- Career in disability services
- Autism-focused practice
- Consulting on accessibility
- Training development
- Academic research

Maria's advocacy journey began small—correcting autism misconceptions in conversations. Energized by impact, she started blogging about adult diagnosis. Reader responses led to local support group creation. Now she balances part-time job with autism consultation, having found sustainable advocacy level. Her rule: advocacy cannot exceed 30% of total energy to prevent burnout.

Sustainable Advocacy Principles

Start Small: One conversation, one post, one action **Honor Capacity**: Advocacy shouldn't harm your wellbeing **Take Breaks**: Regular advocacy sabbaticals prevent burnout **Share the Load**: Collective action over individual heroics **Celebrate Small Wins**: System change happens slowly **Maintain Boundaries**: You can't save everyone

Finding Your Advocacy Niche

Match advocacy to strengths:

- Writers create resources
- Speakers do presentations
- Organizers build programs
- Researchers generate evidence
- Artists change perceptions
- Techies build tools

Tom combines software engineering skills with advocacy by creating apps for autistic adults. His executive function app helps thousands manage daily tasks. This strength-based advocacy feels energizing rather than draining, allowing sustained contribution.

Chapter FAQ: "What does my future look like?"

Your future as an autistic adult can be fulfilling, meaningful, and authentically yours. While specific paths vary, common elements create positive futures:

Acceptance replaces masking: Future energy goes toward growth rather than hiding. Relationships become authentic. Work aligns with strengths. Daily life honors your needs.

Support enables independence: True independence includes appropriate support. Future networks might include professional services, assistive technology, community connections, and mutual aid relationships.

Accommodations are normal: Future workplaces, homes, and relationships incorporate accommodations naturally. Sensory needs, communication differences, and executive function supports become routine rather than special requests.

Community provides belonging: Isolation transforms into connection. Other autistic adults offer understanding impossible from neurotypical relationships alone. Online and offline communities provide mirrors for your experiences.

Interests flourish: Special interests receive time and respect rather than suppression. They might become careers, provide community connections, or simply bring joy. Future schedules protect interest time.

Health improves: Understanding autism allows appropriate healthcare. Burnout decreases with sustainable routines. Mental health improves without constant masking. Physical health benefits from reduced stress.

Contributions matter: Your unique perspective adds value. Maybe through career achievements, creative works, community building, or simply modeling authentic autistic living. Future contributions honor your capabilities.

Daniel, diagnosed at 35, describes his transformation: "I spent three decades exhausted from pretending. Now at 42, I work part-time from home in a field matching my interests. My partner understands my needs. I have autistic friends who get me. My home is sensory heaven. I stopped trying to be neurotypical and started being successfully autistic. It's not perfect—I still face barriers and discrimination. But I'm living as myself for the first time."

Your future won't match neurotypical templates—it will be distinctly, wonderfully autistic. That's not settling for less; it's creating more authentic existence.

Key Takeaways

- Long-term support needs require honest assessment and multi-layered planning
- Financial planning must account for employment variability and support costs
- Healthcare directives should explicitly address autism-related needs
- Sustainable routines balance structure with flexibility
- Advocacy contributions should match capacity to prevent burnout
- Autistic futures can be fulfilling while looking different from neurotypical paths
- Planning should honor your needs rather than force neurotypical standards

Your Handbook Continues

This handbook ends, but your journey continues. You now have frameworks for understanding your past, navigating your present, and planning your future as an autistic adult. Use what serves you; adapt what needs adjusting; discard what doesn't fit. Your autism is uniquely yours—your path forward will be too.

The most radical act may be simply living authentically autistic in a world demanding conformity. By refusing to break yourself fitting into spaces not designed for you, by insisting on accommodations enabling you to thrive, by building life around your actual needs rather than imposed expectations—you create possibility for every autistic person who follows.

Your story matters. Your struggles are valid. Your needs are legitimate. Your future is yours to create.

Welcome to your autistic adulthood. You belong here.

Appendix A: Diagnostic Worksheets

These worksheets serve as practical tools for organizing your thoughts, experiences, and observations before seeking professional assessment. They help you articulate what might feel like scattered experiences into coherent patterns that diagnosticians can understand. Use them as living documents—add to them as memories surface or new patterns emerge.

Childhood History Questionnaire

This questionnaire helps reconstruct your developmental history, often the most challenging aspect of adult diagnosis. Many autistic adults struggle to recall childhood details or had experiences dismissed by caregivers. Answer what you can; gaps in memory are themselves informative.

Early Development (Ages 0-5)

Communication patterns in your earliest years often reveal autistic traits that became masked later:

- Did you speak early, late, or on typical schedule? Some autistic children speak early with advanced vocabulary, while others experience delays
- Did you engage in echolalia—repeating words, phrases, or entire conversations? This might have been dismissed as "cute" or "annoying"
- How did you respond to your name being called? Many autistic children appeared deaf despite normal hearing
- Did you use pronouns correctly, or refer to yourself in third person?
- Were there specific phrases or scripts you used repeatedly?

Play behaviors during early childhood provide diagnostic clues:

- Did you line up toys rather than play imaginatively? This organizational play is common in autistic children
- Were you intensely attached to specific objects? Beyond typical comfort items, this might include unusual attachments
- How did you interact with other children? Parallel play, observing rather than joining, or complete disinterest are common patterns
- Did you engage in repetitive play scenarios? Acting out the same scene repeatedly brings predictability
- Were your interests unusually intense for your age? Memorizing facts about specific topics beyond typical childhood fascination

Sensory experiences shape autistic childhoods profoundly:

- Were you described as "fussy" or "particular" about clothing, food, or environment?
- Did you seek or avoid certain sensory experiences intensely? Spinning, rocking, or avoiding touch
- How did you respond to loud noises, bright lights, or strong smells?
- Were there textures you absolutely couldn't tolerate?
- Did you have unusual sleep patterns or difficulties?

School Age (6-12)

Academic and social experiences during elementary years reveal adaptation patterns:

- How did you perform academically versus socially? Many autistic children show this split
- Did teachers comment on unusual behaviors in reports? "Daydreaming," "in their own world," "needs to focus"
- Were you bullied or excluded? For what reasons?
- Did you have one intense friend rather than friend groups?

- How did you handle changes in routine or teachers?

Learning differences beyond traditional academic struggles:

- Did you interpret instructions literally, missing implied meanings?
- Were group projects particularly challenging?
- Did you excel in systematic subjects (math, spelling) while struggling with interpretive ones?
- How did you handle open-ended assignments?
- Were there subjects you either mastered completely or couldn't grasp at all?

Adolescence (13-18)

Teenage years often mark increased masking and social struggles:

- How did puberty affect your sensory sensitivities and social understanding?
- Did you study social interactions like academic subjects? Many autistic teens consciously learn social rules
- Were you accused of being "weird," "intense," or "different"?
- How did you handle increased social complexity in high school?
- Did you develop special interests that consumed significant time?

Mental health during adolescence provides diagnostic information:

- When did anxiety or depression first appear? These often emerge as masking becomes unsustainable
- Did you experience what you now recognize as meltdowns or shutdowns?

- Were there periods of complete exhaustion or withdrawal?
- How did you cope with overwhelming situations?
- Were there self-harm behaviors or eating difficulties?

Current Challenges Inventory

This inventory helps identify present-day struggles that might stem from unaccommodated autism. Rate each area's impact on your daily life, noting specific examples.

Social Communication Challenges

Interpersonal interactions require constant translation between autistic and neurotypical communication styles:

- Difficulty reading between lines or understanding implied meanings
- Taking statements literally when metaphorical meaning was intended
- Struggling with small talk or "meaningless" social exchanges
- Missing social cues others seem to catch naturally
- Difficulty maintaining "appropriate" eye contact
- Challenges with phone calls or video chats
- Exhaustion after social interactions requiring recovery time

Example descriptions help clarify: "After team meetings, I need 30 minutes alone to recover. I replay conversations trying to understand what people really meant versus what they said."

Executive Function Difficulties

Daily life management challenges that seem disproportionate to your intelligence:

- Starting tasks without external pressure or deadlines
- Switching between activities, especially when deeply focused
- Managing multiple competing priorities simultaneously
- Keeping track of time during activities
- Organizing physical and digital spaces effectively
- Following through on multi-step processes
- Making decisions, especially with multiple options

Specific examples illuminate patterns: "I can design complex software systems but forget to eat lunch daily. My apartment has organizational systems that others find excessive but help me function."

Sensory Processing Differences

Sensory experiences that significantly impact daily functioning:

- Clothing restrictions due to texture, tags, or seams
- Food limitations beyond typical preferences
- Strong reactions to sounds others don't notice
- Light sensitivity affecting work or social environments
- Difficulty filtering background noise in conversations
- Physical reactions to certain smells or visual patterns
- Need for specific pressure, movement, or temperature

Document impact levels: "Fluorescent lights cause headaches within 20 minutes. I wear sunglasses indoors despite social judgment because functioning matters more than appearing normal."

Routine and Change Management

How predictability needs affect your life:

- Distress when routines are disrupted unexpectedly
- Need for detailed advance planning

- Difficulty with spontaneous activities
- Anxiety around travel or new environments
- Specific rituals that must be completed
- Extreme reactions to minor changes
- Recovery time needed after disruptions

Real examples demonstrate impact: "When my morning routine is interrupted, the entire day feels off-balance. I arrive at work 45 minutes early to avoid variable traffic stress."

Sensory Profile Worksheet

This detailed sensory profile helps identify patterns across all sensory systems. Understanding your sensory needs enables better self-advocacy and environment modification.

Auditory (Sound)

Map your sound sensitivities and preferences:

Painful/Overwhelming Sounds:

- Specific frequencies that cause physical discomfort
- Volume levels that others tolerate but you cannot
- Sudden sounds that trigger startles or shutdowns
- Layered sounds (multiple conversations, music plus talking)
- Mechanical sounds (fans, refrigerators, electronics)

Helpful/Regulating Sounds:

- White, pink, or brown noise preferences
- Specific music that aids concentration
- Nature sounds or silence needs
- Repetitive sounds that soothe
- Sound tools used for regulation

Example profile: "High-pitched sounds like children screaming cause immediate fight-or-flight response. I use brown noise apps constantly. Silence is regulation, not emptiness—I can hear electricity humming in 'quiet' rooms."

Visual

Light and visual input significantly impact autistic nervous systems:

Challenging Visual Input:

- Fluorescent or LED lighting reactions
- Bright sunlight sensitivity
- Flashing or strobing effects
- Busy patterns causing disorientation
- Screen brightness tolerance
- Color sensitivities

Supportive Visual Input:

- Preferred lighting types and levels
- Colors that calm or energize
- Visual stims (lava lamps, spinning objects)
- Organization systems reducing visual clutter
- Natural light preferences

Tactile (Touch)

Touch sensitivities affect everything from clothing to relationships:

Difficult Textures/Sensations:

- Clothing materials you cannot tolerate
- Tags, seams, or construction details
- Light touch versus deep pressure preferences

- Temperature sensitivities
- Wet or sticky sensations
- Hair or skin sensitivities

Comforting Touch:

- Weighted blankets or compression
- Specific fabric preferences
- Self-soothing touch behaviors
- Temperature regulation needs
- Movement for proprioceptive input

Gustatory/Olfactory (Taste/Smell)

Food and scent sensitivities impact nutrition and environment navigation:

Challenging Tastes/Smells:

- Food textures you cannot tolerate
- Flavor sensitivities or restrictions
- Scents triggering nausea or headaches
- Cleaning product reactions
- Perfume or cosmetic sensitivities

Safe Foods/Scents:

- Consistent safe foods list
- Preferred preparation methods
- Calming or organizing scents
- Texture preferences
- Temperature requirements

Communication Preferences Chart

This chart helps others understand how to communicate effectively with you across different contexts and energy levels.

Optimal Communication Conditions

When functioning well, these communication methods work best:

- Written versus verbal preferences for different topics
- Processing time needed before responding
- Direct versus indirect communication styles
- Literal versus figurative language tolerance
- Eye contact comfort levels
- Physical positioning preferences

Example entry: "For work discussions, I prefer email with 24-hour response time. For emotional topics, I need written format to process accurately. Video calls drain energy 3x faster than in-person meetings."

Low Energy/Stress Modifications

When stressed, overwhelmed, or in burnout, communication needs change:

- Reduced verbal capacity indicators
- Alternative communication methods needed
- Simplified language requirements
- Response time extensions
- Environmental modifications
- Support person involvement

Crisis Communication Plans

During meltdowns, shutdowns, or medical emergencies:

- Nonverbal communication strategies
- Pre-written cards or digital options
- Trusted person contact information
- Key medical information

- Sensory needs during crisis
- Recovery requirements

Sample crisis card: "I am autistic and temporarily nonverbal. I am not being defiant or rude. Please communicate in writing. I need quiet space and time. Contact: [trusted person]."

Appendix B: Communication Scripts

Pre-written scripts reduce cognitive load during challenging conversations. Customize these templates for your specific situations, voice, and relationships.

Disclosure Scripts for Various Situations

Disclosure scripts provide frameworks for sharing your autism diagnosis strategically. Each script serves different relationship contexts and disclosure goals.

Intimate Partner/Close Family Disclosure

For those closest to you, fuller disclosure often strengthens relationships:

"I need to share something important about myself. I recently discovered I'm autistic. This doesn't change who I am—it explains who I've always been.

All those times I needed exact plans, got overwhelmed at parties, or seemed 'too sensitive'? Those are autistic traits. My brain processes information differently, which affects how I communicate, handle sensory input, and manage daily life.

This diagnosis helps me understand why certain things are harder for me than others. It also means I can better explain my needs and find strategies that actually work. I'm sharing this because I trust you and want you to understand me better.

I know you might have questions or preconceptions about autism. I'm happy to talk more about what this means for me specifically, or I can share some resources that helped me understand. What would be most helpful for you?"

Workplace Disclosure for Accommodations

Professional disclosure focuses on function over diagnosis:

"I'm reaching out regarding some workplace accommodations that would help me perform more effectively. I have a neurological condition that affects sensory processing and communication.

Specifically, I work best with:

- Written instructions for new tasks
- Advance notice of meeting agendas
- Permission to use noise-canceling headphones
- Email communication when possible over phone calls

These simple adjustments would significantly improve my productivity and work quality. I have medical documentation supporting these needs and am happy to work with HR on formal accommodation requests.

Thank you for considering these modifications. I'm committed to contributing my best work and believe these supports will help me do so."

Social Disclosure to Acquaintances

Casual disclosure requires briefer explanation:

"Just so you know, I'm autistic, which means I process things a bit differently. Sometimes I might miss social cues or need things explained directly. If I seem awkward or miss something, just let me know clearly—I appreciate direct communication!"

Medical Provider Disclosure

Healthcare settings require specific information:

"I'm autistic, which affects how I process information and handle medical environments. This means:

- I may need extra processing time for questions
- Fluorescent lights and medical smells can be overwhelming
- I interpret language literally, so please be specific
- I might not show pain or distress in typical ways
- Written instructions help me remember information

Please note this in my chart for future visits. These accommodations help me participate more effectively in my healthcare."

Accommodation Request Templates

Formal accommodation requests require specific language and structure. These templates provide starting points for various contexts.

Educational Accommodation Request

Subject: Request for Academic Accommodations

Dear [Disability Services Coordinator],

I am writing to request academic accommodations for autism spectrum disorder. I have provided diagnostic documentation from [provider name] dated [date].

Based on my disability-related needs, I am requesting the following accommodations:

1. Extended time (1.5x) for exams due to processing speed differences
2. Reduced distraction testing environment due to sensory sensitivities

3. Permission to record lectures for processing verbal information
4. Written instructions for all assignments to accommodate literal thinking
5. Flexibility in group project participation due to social communication challenges

These accommodations address specific barriers I face due to autism while maintaining academic standards. I am happy to discuss implementation details or provide additional documentation as needed.

Thank you for your assistance in ensuring equal access to education.

Sincerely, [Your name]

Workplace Accommodation Request

Dear [HR Representative/Supervisor],

Per the Americans with Disabilities Act, I am requesting reasonable accommodations for autism spectrum disorder. These accommodations would enable me to perform essential job functions more effectively.

Requested accommodations:

Environmental:

- Desk location away from high-traffic areas
- Permission to use noise-canceling headphones
- Adjustment to lighting (desk lamp versus overhead fluorescents)

Communication:

- Written follow-up to verbal instructions
- Meeting agendas provided in advance
- Option to turn off camera during video calls

Schedule:

- Consistent work hours when possible
- Advance notice of schedule changes
- Short breaks for sensory regulation

I believe these modifications would significantly improve my productivity without causing undue hardship. I have medical documentation available and am happy to engage in the interactive process to find mutually beneficial solutions.

Best regards, [Your name]

Boundary-Setting Phrases

Clear boundaries protect autistic wellbeing. These phrases communicate limits respectfully but firmly.

Energy Boundaries

- "I need to limit social events to one per week to maintain my health."
- "I can participate for the first hour, then I'll need to leave."
- "Evening events don't work for me—could we meet earlier?"
- "I need a day to recover after social gatherings, so I won't be available Sunday."

Communication Boundaries

- "I respond better to text than phone calls. Can we communicate that way?"

- "I need 24 hours to process before discussing emotional topics."
- "Please be direct with me—I don't pick up on hints."
- "I'm not ignoring you; I just need processing time."

Sensory Boundaries

- "I can't eat at restaurants with fluorescent lighting. Could we go somewhere else?"
- "Please don't wear strong fragrances around me—they trigger migraines."
- "I need advance warning before physical contact."
- "That texture is painful for me. I need an alternative."

Social Boundaries

- "Small talk exhausts me. I prefer deeper conversations or comfortable silence."
- "I care about you, but I can't handle surprise visits."
- "Group events overwhelm me. Could we meet one-on-one instead?"
- "I need to know the plan in advance. Spontaneous changes cause me distress."

Medical Appointment Preparation

Medical appointments challenge many autistic adults. Preparation scripts ensure important information gets communicated despite stress.

Pre-Appointment Preparation Card

Create a card with essential information:

"I am autistic. This affects my medical visits in these ways:

- I may become nonverbal when stressed

- I process information literally—please avoid metaphors
- I need extra time to process questions
- Fluorescent lights and medical smells are overwhelming
- I may not show pain in typical ways
- Written instructions help me remember information

Please speak directly to me, not my support person. Allow extra time for processing. Thank you for accommodating my needs."

Symptom Description Scripts

Describing symptoms accurately challenges literal thinking:

"I've prepared a written list of my symptoms with specific examples:

- The pain started [specific date]
- On a scale of 1-10, it rates [number]
- It feels like [specific description without metaphors]
- These activities make it worse: [list]
- These help: [list]
- It interferes with these daily activities: [specific examples]"

Question-Asking Framework

Prepare questions in advance:

- "What exactly will this procedure involve?"
- "How long will each step take?"
- "What sensory experiences should I expect?"
- "What are the specific side effects?"
- "Can you write down the important points?"
- "What should I do if [specific concern]?"

Appendix C: Resources Directory

This directory connects you with organizations, communities, and tools supporting autistic adults. Resources focus on autistic-led initiatives providing genuine support rather than cure-focused approaches.

Professional Organizations

Autistic Self Advocacy Network (ASAN)

- Website: autisticadvocacy.org
- Focus: Policy advocacy, resource creation, community building
- Resources: Toolkits, position papers, advocacy guides
- Why helpful: Autistic-led organization centering autistic voices

Autistic Women & Nonbinary Network (AWN)

- Website: awnnetwork.org
- Focus: Gender-specific autistic experiences and advocacy
- Resources: Articles, community forums, resource lists
- Why helpful: Addresses intersection of autism and gender

Academic Autistic Spectrum Partnership in Research and Education (AASPIRE)

- Website: aaspire.org
- Focus: Collaborative research including autistic adults
- Resources: Healthcare toolkits, research findings
- Why helpful: Evidence-based resources created with autistic input

International Association for Autism Research (INSAR)

- Focus: Promoting autism research including autistic researchers
- Resources: Conference presentations, research updates
- Why helpful: Increasing autistic involvement in research

Online Communities

Reddit Communities

- r/AutisticAdults: General adult discussions
- r/AutismInWomen: Gender-specific experiences
- r/autisticpride: Neurodiversity celebration
- r/aspergirls: Women and femme-focused

Facebook Groups

- "Autistic Adults International"
- "Actually Autistic Adults"
- "Autism Late Diagnosis Support and Education"
- Search "[Your City] Autistic Adults" for local groups

Discord Servers

- Autistic Adults server
- Neurodivergent Universe
- Actually Autistic Gamers
- Special interest-specific servers

Other Platforms

- Wrong Planet forums
- The Thinking Person's Guide to Autism
- Autistic Not Weird community
- #ActuallyAutistic Twitter/Instagram communities

Recommended Books and Websites

Books by Autistic Authors

Neurotribes by Steve Silberman

- Comprehensive autism history
- Challenges deficit model
- Promotes neurodiversity understanding

Loud Hands: Autistic People, Speaking

- Anthology of autistic voices
- Diverse perspectives and experiences
- Challenges stereotypes

The Reason I Jump by Naoki Higashida

- Nonverbal autistic perspective
- Challenges assumptions about communication
- Insight into different presentations

Helpful Websites

Autistic Hoya (autistichoya.net)

- Lydia X. Z. Brown's advocacy blog
- Intersectional autism perspectives
- Resource compilations

Neuroclastic (neuroclastic.com)

- Articles by autistic writers
- Practical life guides
- Current autism discussions

Thinking Person's Guide to Autism

- Evidence-based information
- Autistic and parent perspectives
- Resource reviews

Apps and Tools

Communication Apps

- Proloquo2Go: Comprehensive AAC
- Emergency Chat: Temporary speech loss
- Predictable: Text-to-speech

Executive Function Apps

- Todoist: Task management
- Forest: Focus maintenance
- Routinery: Routine guidance
- Time Timer: Visual time tracking

Sensory Regulation Apps

- Noisli: Background noise generation
- Calm: Meditation and sleep stories
- Soothing Sounds: Nature audio

Social Skills Apps

- Social Stories Creator
- Model Me Going Places
- Conversation Builder

Crisis Resources

Mental Health Crisis Lines

- National Suicide Prevention Lifeline: 988
- Crisis Text Line: Text HOME to 741741

- SAMHSA National Helpline: 1-800-662-4357

Autism-Specific Crisis Resources

- Autism Crisis Support Guide (ASAN)
- Autistic Burnout Prevention Toolkit
- Local autism emergency registries

Online Crisis Support

- Autistic peer support crisis groups
- 24/7 autism community forums
- Crisis planning templates

Appendix D: Quick Reference Guides

These condensed guides provide rapid access to key information during challenging moments or for sharing with others.

Common Autistic Traits Checklist

Communication Differences

- ☐ Taking language literally
- ☐ Difficulty with implied meanings
- ☐ Detailed, precise communication style
- ☐ Challenges with small talk
- ☐ Processing delays in conversation
- ☐ Echolalia or scripting
- ☐ Selective mutism during stress

Sensory Processing

- ☐ Over or under-sensitivity to light
- ☐ Sound sensitivity or auditory processing differences
- ☐ Texture aversions (food, clothing, touch)
- ☐ Strong reactions to smells
- ☐ Vestibular or proprioceptive needs
- ☐ Sensory seeking or avoiding behaviors
- ☐ Sensory overload leading to shutdown

Social Differences

- ☐ Difficulty reading social cues
- ☐ Preference for parallel activities
- ☐ Intense, focused friendships
- ☐ Social exhaustion requiring recovery
- ☐ Different empathy expression
- ☐ Challenges with eye contact
- ☐ Misunderstanding of social hierarchies

Repetitive Behaviors and Interests

- ☐ Stimming (rocking, flapping, spinning)
- ☐ Intense special interests
- ☐ Need for routine and predictability
- ☐ Distress at unexpected changes
- ☐ Repetitive play or activities
- ☐ Collecting or organizing objects
- ☐ Echolalia or phrase repetition

Cognitive Patterns

- ☐ Detail-focused thinking
- ☐ Pattern recognition abilities
- ☐ Black-and-white thinking
- ☐ Difficulty with abstract concepts
- ☐ Strong sense of justice
- ☐ Exceptional memory for interests
- ☐ Executive function challenges

Masking Behaviors Identifier

Common Masking Strategies

- Rehearsing conversations in advance
- Copying others' body language and expressions
- Forcing eye contact despite discomfort
- Suppressing stims in public
- Creating "social scripts" for interactions
- Developing different personas for different contexts
- Studying social rules like academic subjects

Signs You're Masking

- Exhaustion after social interactions
- Feeling like you're "performing" rather than being

- Different people know completely different versions of you
- Delayed emotional reactions after events
- Need for extensive alone time to recover
- Loss of authentic self
- Increased anxiety and depression

Masking Costs

- Autistic burnout from sustained effort
- Identity confusion
- Delayed diagnosis
- Mental health impacts
- Physical health effects from stress
- Relationship difficulties
- Loss of authentic connections

Burnout Warning Signs

Early Warning Signs

- Increased sensory sensitivity
- Executive function decline
- Social withdrawal beginning
- Disrupted sleep patterns
- Appetite changes
- Increased stimming
- Communication becoming harder

Escalating Signs

- Simple tasks becoming impossible
- Emotional regulation failing
- Meltdowns increasing
- Physical symptoms appearing
- Complete social withdrawal
- Self-care declining

- Work/school performance dropping

Crisis Signs

- Complete shutdown
- Loss of speech
- Inability to perform basic tasks
- Severe depression/anxiety
- Self-harm thoughts
- Complete routine disruption
- Need for immediate support

Recovery Strategies

- Reduce all optional demands
- Increase sensory regulation
- Prioritize special interests
- Sleep and nutrition focus
- Minimal social contact
- Professional support
- Time—recovery takes time

Self-Advocacy Tips

Know Your Rights

- Workplace accommodations under ADA
- Educational accommodations under Section 504
- Healthcare communication access
- Housing modifications
- Public accommodation requirements

Documentation Strategies

- Keep written records of all requests
- Save email communications
- Document discrimination incidents

- Maintain medical records
- Create accommodation portfolios

Communication Techniques

- Use clear, direct language
- Put requests in writing
- Provide specific examples
- Offer solutions, not just problems
- Know when to escalate
- Build support networks

Building Confidence

- Practice scripts in advance
- Start with small requests
- Celebrate advocacy wins
- Learn from each experience
- Connect with other advocates
- Remember your worth

Sensory Regulation Techniques

Quick Regulation (Under 1 minute)

- Deep pressure: self-hugs, wall pushes
- Movement: rocking, bouncing, spinning
- Breathing: box breathing, extended exhales
- Temperature: cold water, ice cubes
- Oral: chewing gum, crunchy snacks
- Visual: looking at calming images

Medium Regulation (5-15 minutes)

- Weighted blanket or lap pad use
- Listening to regulatory music/sounds
- Progressive muscle relaxation

- Sensory bath or shower
- Organized movement routine
- Special interest engagement

Deep Regulation (30+ minutes)

- Full sensory routine
- Extended special interest time
- Nature immersion
- Creative expression
- Physical exercise
- Complete environment control

Emergency Regulation

- Pre-made sensory kit
- Noise-canceling headphones
- Sunglasses for light
- Familiar scent or taste
- Comfort object
- Safe space retreat

Glossary of Terms

A

AAC (Augmentative and Alternative Communication): Communication methods that supplement or replace speech, including picture cards, sign language, communication apps, and speech-generating devices. Used temporarily during shutdowns or permanently for nonspeaking autistic individuals.

ABLE Account: Tax-advantaged savings account for individuals with disabilities, allowing savings without affecting government benefit eligibility. Must have disability onset before age 26.

Ableism: Discrimination and social prejudice against people with disabilities based on the belief that typical abilities are superior. Includes both systemic barriers and individual attitudes.

Accommodation: Modification or adjustment that enables equal access and participation. Examples include noise-canceling headphones at work, extended test time, or written instructions instead of verbal.

ADA (Americans with Disabilities Act): U.S. federal law prohibiting discrimination based on disability in employment, public accommodations, transportation, and telecommunications.

ADHD (Attention Deficit Hyperactivity Disorder): Neurodevelopmental condition often co-occurring with autism (50-70% of autistic people), affecting attention, hyperactivity, and impulsivity.

Adult Diagnosis: Autism identification after age 18, often involving unique challenges like established masking patterns, lack of childhood records, and identity reconstruction.

Advance Directive: Legal document specifying medical treatment preferences if unable to communicate, particularly important for autistic adults who may become nonverbal during medical stress.

Advocacy: Acting to promote, protect, or support autism acceptance and autistic rights, ranging from personal boundary-setting to systemic change efforts.

AFAB/AMAB: Assigned Female/Male At Birth, relevant because autism presents differently based on socialization and gender expectations.

Alexithymia: Difficulty identifying, describing, or distinguishing emotions, affecting approximately 50% of autistic people. Not lack of emotions but challenge in recognizing them.

Allistic: Non-autistic person, preferred term in neurodiversity movement over "normal" or "typical."

Anxiety Disorders: Mental health conditions occurring in up to 40% of autistic adults, often stemming from navigating non-accommodating environments.

AQ (Autism Spectrum Quotient): Screening tool measuring autistic traits, not diagnostic but useful for self-assessment before seeking formal evaluation.

ARFID (Avoidant/Restrictive Food Intake Disorder): Eating pattern common in autism involving extreme food selectivity due to sensory issues, not related to body image.

ASAN (Autistic Self Advocacy Network): Leading autistic-run organization promoting acceptance, inclusion, and self-determination for autistic people.

Asperger's Syndrome: Outdated diagnostic term removed in DSM-5, now part of autism spectrum disorder. Many avoid due to Hans Asperger's Nazi connections.

Assessment: Formal evaluation process for autism diagnosis, may include interviews, observations, cognitive testing, and developmental history.

Assistive Technology: Tools supporting daily functioning, from simple fidgets to complex AAC devices, noise-canceling headphones to scheduling apps.

Auditory Processing: How the brain interprets sounds, often different in autism, affecting ability to filter background noise or process verbal information.

Augmentative Communication: See AAC.

Autism Speaks: Controversial organization criticized by autistic community for cure focus, lack of autistic leadership, and harmful messaging.

Autism Spectrum Disorder (ASD): Current diagnostic term encompassing range of neurodevelopmental differences affecting communication, sensory processing, social interaction, and behavior patterns.

Autistic Burnout: State of physical, emotional, and mental exhaustion from cumulative stress of navigating non-autistic world without adequate support. Characterized by skill loss, increased sensitivity, and decreased functioning.

Autistic Culture: Shared experiences, values, language, and customs within autistic community, including appreciation for direct communication, acceptance of stimming, and celebration of special interests.

Autistic Inertia: Difficulty starting, stopping, or switching tasks, related to executive function differences. Not laziness but neurological difference.

Autistic Joy: Intense positive emotions often experienced through special interests, stimming, or pattern recognition. Natural autistic expression often suppressed by societal expectations.

Autistic Pride: Movement celebrating autism as identity rather than pathology, rejecting cure mentality in favor of acceptance and accommodation.

Autistic Shutdown: Withdrawal response to overwhelming situations, may include loss of speech, reduced movement, or apparent unresponsiveness. Protective mechanism, not willful behavior.

Autistic Space: Physical or social environment designed for autistic comfort—sensory-friendly, direct communication welcomed, stimming accepted.

B

Bilateral Coordination: Using both sides of body together, often challenging in autism, affecting tasks like driving, sports, or crafts.

Binary Thinking: Tendency toward all-or-nothing thought patterns, common in autism. Can be strength in logical analysis but challenging in nuanced situations.

Binaural Beats: Audio frequencies potentially helpful for sensory regulation and focus, though effectiveness varies individually.

Body Doubling: Working alongside another person for task initiation and maintenance, helpful for executive function challenges.

Body Language: Nonverbal communication through gestures, posture, and movement. Often different in autistic people, leading to misinterpretation.

Bottom-Up Thinking: Processing details before seeing whole picture, common autistic cognitive style contrasting with neurotypical top-down processing.

Boundary Setting: Establishing limits on behavior, demands, or sensory input to maintain wellbeing. Essential skill for sustainable autistic living.

Brain Fog: Cognitive dysfunction including confusion, forgetfulness, and mental fatigue, common during burnout or overload.

Burnout: See Autistic Burnout.

C

Camouflaging: Conscious or unconscious suppression of autistic traits to appear neurotypical. See also Masking.

CAT-Q (Camouflaging Autistic Traits Questionnaire): Assessment tool measuring masking behaviors, helpful for adults whose autism is hidden by compensation strategies.

CBT (Cognitive Behavioral Therapy): Common therapy approach requiring adaptation for autistic clients, as standard CBT may invalidate autistic experiences.

Central Auditory Processing Disorder: Difficulty processing auditory information despite normal hearing, commonly co-occurring with autism.

Central Coherence: Cognitive style favoring details over global processing, explaining autistic strengths in pattern detection and challenges with "big picture" thinking.

Change Resistance: Need for predictability and routine, not stubbornness but neurological need for stability in overwhelming world.

Chosen Family: Intentionally created support network beyond biological relations, particularly important for autistic adults facing family rejection or misunderstanding.

Circadian Rhythm: Natural sleep-wake cycle, often disrupted in autism, leading to delayed sleep phase or irregular patterns.

Co-occurring Conditions: Conditions frequently appearing alongside autism: ADHD, anxiety, depression, epilepsy, EDS, GI issues. Not part of autism but more common.

Code Switching: Alternating between different communication styles for different contexts, exhausting for autistic people managing multiple "masks."

Cognitive Empathy: Understanding others' thoughts and perspectives intellectually, often challenging in autism while emotional empathy remains intact.

Cognitive Load: Mental effort required for processing, often higher for autistic people managing sensory input, social translation, and executive function.

Communication Differences: Variations in how autistic people process and express language, including literal interpretation, direct speech, and processing delays.

Comorbidity: Outdated medical term for co-occurring conditions, implies additional pathology rather than recognizing interconnected experiences.

Compensatory Strategies: Techniques developed to manage autistic traits, often unconsciously, enabling function but potentially hiding support needs.

Compliance Training: Harmful intervention teaching automatic obedience, increasing vulnerability to abuse. Includes ABA focused on eliminating autistic traits.

Compression Clothing: Tight-fitting garments providing proprioceptive input for sensory regulation, helpful for some autistic people.

Context Blindness: Difficulty generalizing skills or knowledge across different situations, explaining why autistic people may struggle with "obvious" applications.

Conversational Scripts: Pre-planned responses for common social situations, reducing real-time processing demands.

Coping Mechanisms: Strategies for managing difficulties, may be healthy (stimming, special interests) or harmful (substance use, self-injury).

Criterion A/B: DSM-5 diagnostic criteria categories—A covers social communication, B covers restricted/repetitive behaviors. Both required for diagnosis.

Cross-Neurotype Communication: Interaction between autistic and non-autistic people, often involving mutual misunderstanding (see Double Empathy Problem).

D

DBT (Dialectical Behavior Therapy): Therapy teaching emotional regulation, distress tolerance, interpersonal skills. Often helpful for autistic adults when adapted appropriately.

Deep Pressure: Firm tactile input calming nervous system, achieved through weighted blankets, tight hugs, or compression clothing.

Demand Avoidance: Extreme difficulty meeting demands, even self-imposed ones. See also PDA.

Depression: Mental health condition affecting up to 40% of autistic adults, often resulting from chronic masking, lack of support, or societal barriers.

Developmental Disability: Disability originating before adulthood affecting major life activities. Autism qualifies though many reject deficit-focused framing.

Developmental History: Record of early milestones, behaviors, and challenges, often required for adult autism diagnosis despite recall difficulties.

Diagnosis: Formal identification of autism by qualified professional, providing access to accommodations and services but not required for self-understanding.

Diagnostic Overshadowing: When autism attribution prevents recognition of other conditions or dismisses legitimate health concerns as "just autism."

Direct Communication: Clear, explicit expression of thoughts and needs, natural for many autistic people but often penalized in indirect communication cultures.

Disability Identity: Positive identification with disability community, rejecting shame and embracing accommodation needs.

Disability Rights: Movement ensuring equal access, opportunity, and dignity for disabled people, foundational to autism acceptance.

Disclosure: Sharing autism diagnosis with others, requiring strategic decisions about who, when, and how much information to share.

Double Empathy Problem: Theory that communication difficulties between autistic and neurotypical people are bidirectional, not solely autistic deficit.

DSM-5: Diagnostic and Statistical Manual, Fifth Edition, containing current autism diagnostic criteria combining previous separate diagnoses.

Dual Diagnosis: Having both autism and intellectual disability, or autism and mental health conditions. Term varies by context.

Dynamic Disability: Disability with fluctuating support needs, describing how autism challenges vary with environment, stress, and energy levels.

Dyspraxia: Motor planning difficulty commonly co-occurring with autism, affecting coordination, handwriting, and daily living tasks.

E

Early Intervention: Services for young autistic children, controversial when focused on eliminating autistic traits rather than supporting development.

Eating Differences: Variations in food acceptance, often sensory-based, including ARFID, same-food preferences, or specific preparation requirements.

Echolalia: Repetition of words, phrases, or sounds serving various functions: processing, communication, self-soothing, or joy. Not meaningless behavior.

Echopraxia: Automatic imitation of observed movements, related to different mirror neuron functioning in autism.

Educational Accommodations: Modifications enabling learning access: extended time, quiet testing, note-taking support, assignment clarifications.

Ehlers-Danlos Syndrome (EDS): Connective tissue disorder with high autism co-occurrence, affecting joints, skin, and multiple body systems.

Emotional Dysregulation: Difficulty managing emotional responses proportionate to situations, often from sensory overload or communication frustration.

Emotional Labor: Effort required to manage feelings and expressions for others' comfort, particularly exhausting when masking autism.

Employment Gap: Period without work, common in autistic adults due to burnout, lack of accommodations, or job-seeking challenges.

Energy Accounting: Tracking energy expenditure and restoration to prevent burnout, recognizing autistic people's different energy economics.

Environmental Modifications: Changes to physical space supporting autistic needs: lighting adjustments, noise reduction, organizational systems.

Equality Act: UK legislation protecting against disability discrimination, including autism, in employment, education, and services.

Executive Dysfunction: Challenges with planning, organization, task initiation, and switching. Not laziness but neurological difference.

Executive Function: Cognitive processes managing goal-directed behavior: working memory, cognitive flexibility, inhibitory control, planning.

Eye Contact: Social expectation causing discomfort, pain, or processing interference for many autistic people. Cultural significance varies globally.

F

Face Blindness: See Prosopagnosia.

Fawning: Trauma response involving people-pleasing to avoid conflict, common in autistic people facing repeated social rejection.

Fidget Tools: Objects for sensory regulation through tactile manipulation: stress balls, fidget cubes, thinking putty.

Fight/Flight/Freeze/Fawn: Trauma responses, with freeze and fawn particularly common in autistic people facing overwhelming situations.

Fine Motor Skills: Small muscle movements for tasks like writing, buttoning, or crafts. Often challenging in autism.

Flat Affect: Reduced emotional expression through face or voice, not indicating lack of internal emotion. Often misinterpreted.

Food Aversion: Strong negative response to specific foods, usually sensory-based regarding texture, temperature, taste, or smell.

Formal Diagnosis: Official autism identification by qualified professional, contrasting with self-diagnosis/self-identification.

Functioning Labels: Problematic "high/low functioning" categorizations failing to capture varying support needs across contexts and time.

Functional Communication: Effective information exchange regardless of method—speech, writing, AAC, behavior.

G

Gaslighting: Psychological manipulation making someone question their reality, commonly experienced by autistic people told their perceptions are wrong.

Gaze Aversion: Looking away to improve processing, not rudeness or disinterest. Natural autistic behavior often forcibly "corrected."

Gender Diversity: Higher rates of transgender and non-binary identification among autistic people, possibly from less internalization of social norms.

Genetic Component: Autism's hereditary aspects, with multiple genes involved. Runs in families though presentation varies.

Gestalt Processing: Perceiving whole patterns before details, opposite of typical autistic detail-focused processing.

Gross Motor Skills: Large muscle movements for walking, jumping, balance. Often affected in autism with retained reflexes or coordination challenges.

Group Dynamics: Social interactions in multiple-person settings, exponentially more complex than one-on-one interaction for autistic processing.

H

Habituation: Decreased response to repeated stimuli, often different in autism leading to continued noticing of "background" sensory input.

Hand Flapping: Common stim involving rapid hand movement, often expressing joy or processing emotion. Natural behavior unnecessarily pathologized.

Healthcare Proxy: Designated person making medical decisions when patient cannot, crucial for autistic adults who may lose speech under stress.

Hearing Sensitivity: See Hyperacusis.

Heavy Work: Proprioceptive activities involving muscle resistance: pushing, pulling, carrying. Regulating for sensory seekers.

Hyperfocus: Intense concentration on activity of interest, losing track of time and surroundings. Strength when channeled, challenging when inflexible.

Hyperlexia: Advanced reading ability often with comprehension lag, common in autistic children. May persist as reading/writing strength.

Hypermobility: Excessive joint flexibility common in autism, possibly related to connective tissue differences. Can cause pain and injury.

Hyperacusis: Extreme sensitivity to sounds others tolerate, from painful physical sensation to overwhelming processing demands.

Hyporesponsive: Under-reactive to sensory input, may seek intense experiences or not notice injuries. Varies by sense and situation.

I

Identity-First Language: "Autistic person" rather than "person with autism," preferred by many autistic adults viewing autism as integral identity.

IEP (Individualized Education Program): U.S. special education plan outlining goals and services. Doesn't transfer to college requiring new accommodations.

Impostor Syndrome: Feeling of "faking" autism despite valid diagnosis, common in late-diagnosed adults with strong masking abilities.

Inertia: See Autistic Inertia.

Infodumping: Sharing extensive information about topics of interest, natural autistic communication often misunderstood as lecturing.

Intellectual Disability: Cognitive impairment co-occurring in some autistic people, distinct from autism. Many autistic people have average or above intelligence.

Interoception: Awareness of internal body signals: hunger, thirst, bathroom needs, emotions. Often different in autism affecting self-care.

Internalized Ableism: Absorbed negative beliefs about disability and autism, creating shame and self-rejection requiring conscious unlearning.

Interpersonal Therapy: Therapy focusing on relationships and communication, requires adaptation for autistic communication differences.

Intersectionality: How multiple identities (autistic, race, gender, sexuality, class) interact creating unique experiences and barriers.

J

Joint Attention: Shared focus between people, develops differently in autism. Parallel attention (focusing on same activity separately) may be preferred.

Justice Sensitivity: Strong reaction to unfairness or rule-breaking, common autistic trait leading to advocacy but also distress.

K

Kinesthetic Learning: Learning through movement and doing rather than listening or reading, helpful for many autistic people.

L

Language Delay: Later speech development, previous diagnostic requirement removed in DSM-5 recognizing autism without language delay.

Language Processing: How brain interprets and produces language, often involving longer processing time and literal interpretation in autism.

Late Diagnosis: Autism identification in adulthood, creating unique challenges of unlearning internalized ableism and reconstructing identity.

Learned Helplessness: Psychological state from repeated inability to control environment, risk for autistic people facing constant correction.

Letter Board: Communication tool for spelling messages, controversial due to facilitator influence concerns but effective for some.

Light Sensitivity: Discomfort or pain from lighting, especially fluorescents. May require sunglasses indoors or lighting modifications.

Literal Thinking: Taking language at exact meaning without inferring subtext, natural autistic communication style causing frequent misunderstandings.

Living Will: Document specifying end-of-life care preferences, should include autism-specific needs and communication requirements.

Lost Generation: Adults who reached adulthood before autism awareness expanded, navigating life without understanding or support.

M

Masking: Camouflaging autistic traits to appear neurotypical through conscious or unconscious suppression and performance. Major burnout contributor.

Medical Model: Views autism as disorder requiring treatment or cure, contrasting with neurodiversity paradigm viewing it as natural variation.

Meltdown: Intense external response to overwhelming situation involving crying, yelling, or aggression. Not tantrum but nervous system overload.

Mental Health: Psychological wellbeing, challenged by higher rates of anxiety, depression, and trauma in autistic adults from societal barriers.

Metacognition: Thinking about thinking, including self-monitoring and strategy adjustment. May be different in autism affecting learning approaches.

Mindblindness: Outdated theory claiming autistic people cannot understand others have different thoughts. Replaced by double empathy problem understanding.

Minimal Support Needs: Requiring less daily assistance, though may still need significant accommodations. Replaces problematic "high-functioning" label.

Mirror Neurons: Brain cells activated when observing others' actions, functioning differently in autism affecting automatic mimicry and learning.

Misdiagnosis: Incorrect psychiatric labels before autism recognition: borderline personality disorder, schizophrenia, bipolar disorder, anxiety alone.

Mixed Neurotype: Relationships or groups containing both autistic and non-autistic members, requiring intentional accommodation and understanding.

Monotropism: Attention focused intensely on few interests rather than distributed across many, explaining autistic cognitive style and challenges.

Motor Planning: Organizing and executing movements, often challenging in autism affecting daily tasks despite intact motor ability.

Movement Differences: Variations in gait, posture, gesture use distinguishing autistic movement patterns, not deficits but differences.

Multimodal Communication: Using various methods (speech, writing, AAC, behavior) recognizing communication beyond verbal speech alone.

Mutism: See Selective Mutism.

N

Neurotypical: Person with typical neurological development, not superior to neurodivergent but different. Often shortened to NT.

Neurodiversity: Concept that neurological differences are natural human variations deserving acceptance rather than cure.

Neurodivergent: Umbrella term for people whose neurology differs from typical: autistic, ADHD, dyslexic, etc.

Neuroplasticity: Brain's ability to form new connections, basis for learning and adaptation throughout life including autistic development.

Nonverbal/Nonspeaking: Not using speech to communicate, preferred term nonspeaking as nonverbal implies no communication versus different methods.

Nothing About Us Without Us: Disability rights principle requiring inclusion of affected people in decisions affecting them.

O

Object Permanence: Understanding things exist when not visible, may develop differently in autism affecting organization and relationships.

Occupational Therapy: Therapy supporting daily living skills, sensory integration, and functional abilities. Helpful when neurodiversity-affirming.

Overstimulation: Sensory or information overload exceeding processing capacity, leading to meltdown, shutdown, or urgent escape need.

Overwhelm: State of exceeded capacity from sensory, social, emotional, or cognitive demands. Requires immediate support and reduction.

P

Parallel Play: Engaging in activities alongside others without direct interaction, natural autistic social style persisting into adulthood.

Pathological Demand Avoidance (PDA): Profile involving extreme avoidance of everyday demands, controversial but describing some autistic experiences.

Pattern Recognition: Ability to identify regularities and connections, often heightened in autism contributing to various strengths.

Peer Support: Assistance from others with similar experiences, particularly valuable from other autistic adults understanding lived reality.

Perfectionism: Extremely high personal standards, common in autism from black-and-white thinking and anxiety about "doing it wrong."

Perseveration: Repetitive focus on thoughts or topics, serving emotional regulation or processing functions despite social inconvenience.

Person-First Language: "Person with autism" phrasing, generally rejected by autistic community preferring identity-first language.

Perspective Taking: Understanding others' viewpoints, may be challenging across neurotypes but not absent in autistic people.

Polyvagal Theory: Framework understanding nervous system responses to safety/threat, relevant to autistic sensory and social experiences.

Pragmatic Language: Social use of language including context, nonverbal cues, and implied meaning. Often challenging in autism.

Predictability Need: Requirement for routine and knowing what to expect, providing safety in overwhelming world.

Prevalence: Frequency in population, current estimates 1-2% for autism though likely higher with missed diagnoses.

Processing Delay: Time needed to understand and respond to information, normal autistic variation requiring patience not pressure.

Processing Differences: Variations in how autistic brains handle information: bottom-up, detail-focused, simultaneous multiple channels.

Proprioception: Body position awareness often different in autism, affecting coordination, spatial navigation, and physical comfort.

Prosopagnosia: Face blindness difficulty recognizing faces, more common in autism. Relies on other identification features.

Protest Behaviors: Actions expressing distress or opposition, often mislabeled as "behaviors" when actually communication attempts.

Proxemics: Study of personal space use, often different in autism with unique comfort zones and touch boundaries.

Psychoeducation: Learning about one's condition, crucial for late-diagnosed adults understanding lifelong experiences through autism lens.

Q

Quality of Life: Subjective wellbeing improved more by acceptance and accommodation than by appearing "normal."

R

RAADS-R: Ritvo Autism Asperger Diagnostic Scale-Revised, screening tool particularly useful for identifying masked autism in adults.

Reasonable Accommodation: Modifications enabling equal access without fundamental alteration or undue hardship, legally required in many contexts.

Receptive Language: Understanding others' communication, may be stronger or weaker than expressive language in autism.

Reciprocity: Back-and-forth social exchange, may look different in autism with parallel sharing rather than typical turn-taking.

Recovery Time: Period needed after demanding activities to restore energy and sensory balance, often longer for autistic people.

Rejection Sensitive Dysphoria (RSD): Extreme emotional response to real or perceived rejection, common in ADHD and autism.

Repetitive Behaviors: Actions repeated for regulation, joy, or communication including stimming, routines, and focused interests.

Restricted Interests: Intense focus on specific topics, providing joy, expertise, and emotional regulation. Strength when supported.

Routine Need: Requirement for predictable patterns reducing cognitive load and anxiety in unpredictable world.

S

Safe Foods: Reliably tolerable foods when sensory sensitivities limit options, not pickiness but neurological need.

Sameness Need: Preference for consistency and routine, protective against overwhelming change not rigid defiance.

Scripting: Using memorized phrases for communication, functional strategy reducing real-time language generation demands.

Section 504: U.S. law prohibiting disability discrimination in federally funded programs, providing educational accommodations.

Selective Mutism: Inability to speak in specific situations despite speech ability, common in autistic stress responses.

Self-Advocacy: Communicating one's needs and rights, essential skill for autistic adults navigating non-accommodating systems.

Self-Diagnosis: Identifying as autistic without professional diagnosis, valid in autistic community recognizing barriers to formal assessment.

Self-Regulation: Managing one's emotional and sensory state, achieved through stimming, routines, and environmental control.

Sensory Differences: Variations in processing sensory information, core autism feature affecting daily life across all senses.

Sensory Diet: Planned sensory activities meeting regulation needs throughout day, not food but sensory input planning.

Sensory Integration: How nervous system processes and organizes sensory information, different in autism requiring accommodations.

Sensory Overload: Overwhelming sensory input exceeding processing capacity, causing meltdown, shutdown, or escape need.

Sensory Processing Disorder (SPD): Difficulty processing sensory information, common in autism though not exclusive to it.

Sensory Seeking: Actively pursuing intense sensory experiences for regulation: spinning, jumping, loud music, spicy foods.

Sensory Sensitivity: Heightened awareness and response to sensory input others might not notice or tolerate easily.

Shutdown: Internal withdrawal response to overwhelm, appearing as unresponsiveness, reduced movement, or temporary skill loss.

Social Anxiety: Fear of social judgment, common in autistic people from repeated negative experiences and communication challenges.

Social Camouflaging: See Masking.

Social Communication: Exchange of information in social contexts, involving verbal and nonverbal elements challenging in autism.

Social Model of Disability: Framework locating disability in societal barriers rather than individual deficits, foundational to neurodiversity movement.

Social Motivation: Desire for social connection, present in many autistic people despite different expression and interaction preferences.

Social Skills Training: Teaching neurotypical social rules, controversial when forcing masking rather than mutual understanding.

Special Interest: Intense, focused passion providing joy, expertise, emotional regulation, and identity. Not obsession but strength.

Spoon Theory: Metaphor for limited energy requiring careful allocation, relevant to autistic energy management needs.

SSDI/SSI: U.S. disability benefits providing financial support, though application process challenging for autistic adults.

Stereotypy: Clinical term for repetitive movements, stigmatizing natural autistic stimming behaviors.

Stimming: Self-stimulatory behavior for regulation, expression, or joy. Includes rocking, flapping, spinning, vocal sounds. Natural and necessary.

Strengths-Based Approach: Focusing on autistic abilities and interests rather than deficits, promoting genuine development and wellbeing.

Support Needs: Assistance required for daily living, varying across contexts and time. More accurate than functioning labels.

Synesthesia: Blending of senses (seeing sounds, tasting colors), more common in autistic people enriching sensory experience.

Systematic Thinking: Understanding rule-based patterns and systems, common autistic strength in various fields.

T

Task Switching: Moving between different activities, often requiring significant transition time and energy in autism.

Texting: Written communication often preferred by autistic people for processing time and clarity without nonverbal complexity.

Theory of Mind: Ability to understand others have different thoughts, present in autistic people but may develop differently.

Therapeutic Alliance: Relationship between therapist and client, requiring therapist understanding of autistic communication and needs.

Tics: Involuntary movements or sounds, can co-occur with autism especially with ADHD. Distinguished from voluntary stimming.

Time Agnosia: Difficulty sensing time passage, common in autism affecting scheduling and time management.

Time Blindness: Poor awareness of time passing, different from time agnosia involving attention and executive function.

Toe Walking: Walking on toes rather than flat feet, common in autism from sensory or proprioceptive differences.

Token Economy: Behavioral reward system, controversial in autism for teaching compliance over genuine development.

Traits: Characteristics associated with autism, preferred over "symptoms" which implies disease requiring cure.

Transition Planning: Preparing for changes between activities, life stages, or environments, requiring extra time and support in autism.

Trauma-Informed Care: Treatment recognizing high trauma rates in autistic people from ableism, requiring adapted approaches.

Treatment: In neurodiversity framework, means support and accommodation rather than attempting to cure autism itself.

U

Underdiagnosis: Failure to identify autism, particularly in women, people of color, and older adults due to biased criteria.

Understimulation: Insufficient sensory input causing discomfort, restlessness, or seeking behaviors to meet sensory needs.

Uneven Profile: Significant variation between different skill areas, characteristic of autism. Strengths coexist with support needs.

Universal Design: Creating environments accessible to all, benefiting autistic people through reduced sensory and communication barriers.

Unmasking: Process of reducing camouflaging behaviors, often following diagnosis. Requires safety and may temporarily increase visible traits.

V

Validity: In diagnosis context, whether assessment accurately identifies autism across diverse presentations including masked adults.

Vestibular: Balance and spatial orientation sense, often different in autism affecting movement preferences and tolerances.

Visual Supports: Pictures, schedules, or written instructions supporting understanding and memory, helpful across age ranges.

Visual Thinking: Processing information in images rather than words, common autistic cognitive style with various advantages.

Vocal Stimming: Repetitive sounds, humming, echolalia for regulation or joy. Natural behavior not requiring elimination.

W

Weighted Items: Blankets, vests, or lap pads providing deep pressure for sensory regulation and anxiety reduction.

White Matter: Brain tissue connecting regions, showing differences in autistic brains affecting information integration.

Working Memory: Holding information while using it, often challenged in autism especially with multiple simultaneous demands.

Workplace Accommodations: Modifications enabling job performance: noise reduction, written instructions, scheduling flexibility, sensory breaks.

X

X-linked: Genetic pattern potentially explaining higher male diagnosis rates, though gender bias in diagnosis also significant factor.

Y

Young Adults: Transitional age facing unique challenges moving from pediatric to adult services, often losing supports.

Z

Zone of Regulation: Framework for understanding emotional/sensory states, useful when adapted for autistic experiences versus neurotypical expectations.

Zoning Out: Dissociative response to overwhelm, protective mechanism when environment exceeds processing capacity.

References

1. American Psychiatric Association. (2022). Diagnostic and statistical manual of mental disorders (5th ed., text rev.). American Psychiatric Publishing.
2. Hull, L., Petrides, K. V., & Mandy, W. (2020). The female autism phenotype and camouflaging: A narrative review. Review Journal of Autism and Developmental Disorders, 7(4), 306-317.
3. Fletcher-Watson, S., & Happé, F. (2019). Autism: A new introduction to psychological theory and current debate. Routledge.
4. Brukner-Wertman, Y., Laor, N., & Golan, O. (2016). Social (pragmatic) communication disorder and its relation to the autism spectrum: Dilemmas arising from the DSM-5 classification. Journal of Autism and Developmental Disorders, 46(8), 2821-2829.
5. Pellicano, E., & den Houting, J. (2022). Annual research review: Shifting from 'normal science' to neurodiversity in autism science. Journal of Child Psychology and Psychiatry, 63(4), 381-396.
6. Singer, J. (2017). Neurodiversity: The birth of an idea. Judy Singer.
7. Chapman, R. (2020). The reality of autism: On the metaphysics of disorder and diversity. Philosophical Psychology, 33(6), 799-819.
8. Milton, D. E. (2012). On the ontological status of autism: The 'double empathy problem'. Disability & Society, 27(6), 883-887.
9. Lai, M. C., & Baron-Cohen, S. (2015). Identifying the lost generation of adults with autism spectrum conditions. The Lancet Psychiatry, 2(11), 1013-1027.
10. Courchesne, V., Meilleur, A. A., Poulin-Lord, M. P., Dawson, M., & Soulières, I. (2015). Autistic children at risk of being underestimated: School-based pilot study of a strength-informed assessment. Molecular Autism, 6(1), 1-10.

11. Jaswal, V. K., & Akhtar, N. (2019). Being versus appearing socially uninterested: Challenging assumptions about social motivation in autism. Behavioral and Brain Sciences, 42, e82.
12. Baldwin, S., & Costley, D. (2016). The experiences and needs of female adults with high-functioning autism spectrum disorder. Autism, 20(4), 483-495.
13. Taylor, L. E., Swerdfeger, A. L., & Eslick, G. D. (2014). Vaccines are not associated with autism: An evidence-based meta-analysis of case-control and cohort studies. Vaccine, 32(29), 3623-3629.
14. Kanner, L. (1943). Autistic disturbances of affective contact. Nervous Child, 2(3), 217-250.
15. Asperger, H. (1944). Die "Autistischen Psychopathen" im Kindesalter. Archiv für Psychiatrie und Nervenkrankheiten, 117(1), 76-136.
16. American Psychiatric Association. (1994). Diagnostic and statistical manual of mental disorders (4th ed.). American Psychiatric Publishing.
17. American Psychiatric Association. (2013). Diagnostic and statistical manual of mental disorders (5th ed.). American Psychiatric Publishing.
18. Loomes, R., Hull, L., & Mandy, W. P. L. (2017). What is the male-to-female ratio in autism spectrum disorder? A systematic review and meta-analysis. Journal of the American Academy of Child & Adolescent Psychiatry, 56(6), 466-474.
19. Dean, M., Harwood, R., & Kasari, C. (2017). The art of camouflage: Gender differences in the social behaviors of girls and boys with autism spectrum disorder. Autism, 21(6), 678-689.
20. Begeer, S., Mandell, D., Wijnker-Holmes, B., Venderbosch, S., Rem, D., Stekelenburg, F., & Koot, H. M. (2013). Sex differences in the timing of identification among children and adults with autism spectrum disorders. Journal of Autism and Developmental Disorders, 43(5), 1151-1156.

21. Strang, J. F., Powers, M. D., Knauss, M., Sibarium, E., Leibowitz, S. F., Kenworthy, L., ... & Anthony, L. G. (2018). "They thought it was an obsession": Trajectories and perspectives of autistic transgender and gender-diverse adolescents. Journal of Autism and Developmental Disorders, 48(12), 4039-4055.
22. de Leeuw, A., Happé, F., & Hoekstra, R. A. (2020). A conceptual framework for understanding the cultural and contextual factors on autism across the globe. Autism Research, 13(7), 1029-1050.
23. Mandell, D. S., Wiggins, L. D., Carpenter, L. A., Daniels, J., DiGuiseppi, C., Durkin, M. S., ... & Kirby, R. S. (2009). Racial/ethnic disparities in the identification of children with autism spectrum disorders. American Journal of Public Health, 99(3), 493-498.
24. Lindblom, A. (2014). Under-detection of autism among First Nations children in British Columbia, Canada. Disability & Society, 29(8), 1248-1259.
25. Happé, F. G., & Charlton, R. A. (2012). Aging in autism spectrum disorders: A mini-review. Gerontology, 58(1), 70-78.
26. Howlin, P., & Magiati, I. (2017). Autism spectrum disorder: Outcomes in adulthood. Current Opinion in Psychiatry, 30(2), 69-76.
27. Pearson, A., & Rose, K. (2021). A conceptual analysis of autistic masking: Understanding the narrative of stigma and the illusion of neurotypical adherence. Autism in Adulthood, 3(1), 52-60.
28. Cage, E., & Troxell-Whitman, Z. (2019). Understanding the reasons, contexts and costs of camouflaging for autistic adults. Journal of Autism and Developmental Disorders, 49(5), 1899-1911.
29. Livingston, L. A., Shah, P., & Happé, F. (2019). Compensatory strategies below the behavioural surface in autism: A qualitative study. The Lancet Psychiatry, 6(9), 766-777.

30. Demetriou, E. A., Lampit, A., Quintana, D. S., Naismith, S. L., Song, Y. J. C., Pye, J. E., ... & Guastella, A. J. (2018). Autism spectrum disorders: A meta-analysis of executive function. Molecular Psychiatry, 23(5), 1198-1204.
31. MacLennan, K., Roach, L., & Tavassoli, T. (2020). The relationship between sensory reactivity differences and anxiety subtypes in autistic children. Autism Research, 13(5), 785-795.
32. Hayward, S. M., McVilly, K. R., & Stokes, M. A. (2018). "Always a glass ceiling." Gender or autism; the barrier to occupational inclusion. Research in Autism Spectrum Disorders, 56, 50-60.
33. Baron-Cohen, S., Wheelwright, S., Skinner, R., Martin, J., & Clubley, E. (2001). The autism-spectrum quotient (AQ): Evidence from Asperger syndrome/high-functioning autism, males and females, scientists and mathematicians. Journal of Autism and Developmental Disorders, 31(1), 5-17.
34. Hull, L., Mandy, W., Lai, M. C., Baron-Cohen, S., Allison, C., Smith, P., & Petrides, K. V. (2019). Development and validation of the camouflaging autistic traits questionnaire (CAT-Q). Journal of Autism and Developmental Disorders, 49(3), 819-833.
35. Ritvo, R. A., Ritvo, E. R., Guthrie, D., Ritvo, M. J., Hufnagel, D. H., McMahon, W., ... & Eloff, J. (2011). The Ritvo Autism Asperger Diagnostic Scale-Revised (RAADS-R): A scale to assist the diagnosis of autism spectrum disorder in adults: An international validation study. Journal of Autism and Developmental Disorders, 41(8), 1076-1089.
36. Americans with Disabilities Act of 1990, 42 U.S.C. § 12101 et seq. (1990).
37. Section 504 of the Rehabilitation Act of 1973, 29 U.S.C. § 794 (1973).

38. U.S. Department of Education. (2020). Protecting students with disabilities. Office for Civil Rights. https://www2.ed.gov/about/offices/list/ocr/504faq.html
39. Spain, D., Sin, J., Linder, K. B., McMahon, J., & Happé, F. (2018). Social anxiety in autism spectrum disorder: A systematic review. Research in Autism Spectrum Disorders, 52, 51-68.
40. Bemmouna, D., & Weiner, L. (2023). Linehan's biosocial model applied to emotion dysregulation in autism: A narrative review of the literature and an illustrative case conceptualization. Frontiers in Psychiatry, 14, 1238116.
41. Lai, M. C., Kassee, C., Besney, R., Bonato, S., Hull, L., Mandy, W., ... & Ameis, S. H. (2019). Prevalence of co-occurring mental health diagnoses in the autism population: A systematic review and meta-analysis. The Lancet Psychiatry, 6(10), 819-829.
42. Raymaker, D. M., Teo, A. R., Steckler, N. A., Lentz, B., Scharer, M., Delos Santos, A., ... & Nicolaidis, C. (2020). "Having all of your internal resources exhausted beyond measure and being left with no clean-up crew": Defining autistic burnout. Autism in Adulthood, 2(2), 132-143.
43. Crompton, C. J., Hallett, S., Ropar, D., Flynn, E., & Fletcher-Watson, S. (2020). 'I never realised everybody felt as happy as I do when I am around autistic people': A thematic analysis of autistic adults' relationships with autistic and neurotypical friends and family. Autism, 24(6), 1438-1448.
44. Pecora, L. A., Hancock, G. I., Hooley, M., Demmer, D. H., Attwood, T., Mesibov, G. B., & Stokes, M. A. (2020). Gender identity, sexual orientation and romantic relationships in adolescents and adults with autism spectrum disorder. Autism, 24(7), 1985-1998.
45. Milton, D. E. (2012). On the ontological status of autism: The 'double empathy problem'. Disability & Society, 27(6), 883-887.

46. Cage, E., Di Monaco, J., & Newell, V. (2018). Experiences of autism acceptance and mental health in autistic adults. Journal of Autism and Developmental Disorders, 48(2), 473-484.
47. Eilenberg, J. S., Paff, M., Harrison, A. J., & Long, K. A. (2019). Disparities based on race, ethnicity, and socioeconomic status over the transition to adulthood among adolescents and young adults on the autism spectrum: A systematic review. Current Psychiatry Reports, 21(5), 1-16.
48. Nicolaidis, C., Raymaker, D., Kapp, S. K., Baggs, A., Ashkenazy, E., McDonald, K., ... & Joyce, A. (2019). The AASPIRE practice-based guidelines for the inclusion of autistic adults in research as co-researchers and study participants. Autism, 23(8), 2007-2019.
49. Crane, L., Hearst, C., Ashworth, M., Davies, J., & Hill, E. L. (2021). Supporting newly identified or diagnosed autistic adults: An initial evaluation of an autistic-led programme. Journal of Autism and Developmental Disorders, 51(3), 892-905.

www.ingramcontent.com/pod-product-compliance
Lightning Source LLC
Chambersburg PA
CBHW062155080426
42734CB00010B/1697